Cohn - Visionary Quantum Healing™

Note

Visionary Quantum Healing provides a definitive introduction to a different concept of healing that draws upon new science.

Are you looking for an effective alternative to holistic or modern medicine? Would you like an alternative that requires no belief system but offers instant results? Then look no further. Visionary Quantum Healing teaches you how to use and control your own power for healing yourself and others—in body, mind, and soul.

Visionary Quantum Healing is not a complex system. This book makes it easy for anyone to learn the basic principles even without medical training. Dr. Cohn draws upon his extensive experience in healing to illustrate the dramatic transformations that can occur after just one treatment.

The Complete Guide to Visionary Quantum Healing™

21st Century Healing for the Body, Mind, Heart and Soul

Salomon Cohn, DCH(c), Ph.D.
Visionary Healer

Publisher's Note

Important notice from the publisher and the author:

This book is available to the public with the understanding that neither the publisher nor the author is engaged in rendering psychological, medical, financial, legal, religious, or other professional services. The publisher and the writer cannot be held responsible for actions taken by the individual. Persons choosing to follow the principles and modalities presented here should consult beforehand with their physicians and other competent professional advisors and counselors. Ultimately, you, the reader, must take full responsibility for your health.

Persons choosing to follow principles and modalities presented here should consult beforehand with their physician and other competent professional advisors and counselors.

Some names are either imaginary or are used fictitiously. Any resemblance to actual persons, living or dead, and to events or locations is entirely coincidental.

Library of Congress Cataloging-in-Publication Data:
ISBN 0-9774545-0-9

Dedication

I dedicate this book to the memory of my father, Abraham Albert Cohn;

and to the memory of my mother, Mazal Delouya Pinto Cohn, whose prayers had the healing gift of love. Thank you for recognizing and encouraging my own healing power.

Acknowledgments

I thank GOD, who has always been there for me, especially after my free-fall skydiving accident. Thank you for sending the two angels to save my life once again.

In addition, I wish to thank my son Ari, chiropractor, to my daughter Ilana, film director and actress. Thank you for your love and support and belief in me! I am a proud and blessed father.

Thanks, also to my brothers and sisters in-law, Jacob and Shoshana, Isaac and Silvia, David and Rose, Moses and Shoula, Oury and Shosh, and to my sister and brother-in-law, Rachel and Meyer Levy, and to my 55 nephews and nieces for their unconditional love and support.

Sincere thanks to Paul W. Rea, Ph.D. and Linda Jay Geldens, whose editorial skills truly enhanced the clarity of my message.

Sincere thanks to my friend Mike Doty for his computer skills. I am truly grateful.

Sincere thanks to my dear friend, Mony Vital, Ph.D. for his special friendship, for being a mentor and a source of support at the time of my injury. He was and is greatly appreciated.

Sincere thanks to Judith Schlesinger Fish and

Howard Fish, and to Kenny and Mazal Bordo, for their true friendship, love and support.

Sincere thanks to my colleague, Dr. Rimon Issac, D.O. After receiving one successful treatment from me, we connected, and he has become a great and supportive friend.

Sincere thanks to Helen Tobar for volunteering her time and her patience to serve as a model in some of the book's photographs.

Thanks be to my friends Joseph Schmidt, Angela Mar, Lee and Jenny Chung, Dr. Carol Lewis, Ph.D., Salomon and Ester Ovadia, Bernard and Peggy Moizel, Joseph and Seija Moizel, Marco and Rivka Porat, David, Beny, and Susan Bouskila, Ann Hernandez, Paul Rosen, Ph.D., David Webster MD, Shoula Ben Simon, Elias and Tina Shamash, Rami and Sima Cohen, Roger and Sara Ashkenazy, David Ohana, Oury and Ester Zemak, Avi and Jacky Shalem, Abraham Magidish, Bobby and Mira Coluccio, Joe and Hila Rosha, Jack and Elena Shamash, Joseph Langer, Simon Barzelay, Patricio and Ester Martinez, Cesar and Jenny Salas, Franco and Margarita Alessi, Zion and Jewel Shlomi, Marchelo and Helen Tobar, Efy and Sherlly Khalfy, Rabbi Shalom and Ora Ezran, David and Nena Betsallel, Joe and Rika Hahn Sternlib, Dr. Jeanne N Schurz, Ph.D., Herbert and Zelina Soffer, Carlos and Lucy Porac, with whom I have been blessed, and who have been there supporting me through my recovery.

Foreword

I first met Salomon Cohn in September 2003, in response to a call to assist him with his computer. At the time I had a chronically sore hand from carpal tunnel which was aggravated by working on the computer. Salomon gave me a Visionary Quantum Healing treatment, after which, the pain stayed away. A year later, Salomon gave me another healing treatment because I had been feeling sluggish, and had no vitality. Soon after the treatment, I reached a state of cheerfulness and energy comparable to the way I had felt ten years earlier. My whole outlook in life, and even my family relationships, improved. The treatment also enabled me to work better with my clients by getting to the bottom of their issues and problems faster.

The VQH treatment, which I had in Salomon's clinic, took just twenty minutes. I was mesmerized by the elegance and power of the intervention that Salomon demonstrated. I am sold on VQH and look forward to studying the process and attending an upcoming seminar given by Salomon.

What distinguishes *The Complete Guide to Visionary Quantum Healing* is the depth of study Salomon brings to his writing. Here is a man whose library of healing books includes every significant work in the field. He's read them all! That's very important, since most people with a healing background only study the work of one school of thought. As you'll learn from this book, Salomon has studied the development of alternative medicine from its inception thousands of years ago in Egypt and India to the wisdom of the Hebrew Kabbalah and Scripture, to twentieth-century masters such as Carl Jung, Richard Gerber, and James Gleick.

Salomon has taken complex and diverse concepts and distilled them to their essence, making them simple to learn, understand, and use. This book is an excellent introductory text for clients, students, and practitioners just beginning to study the art and science of Visionary Quantum Healing.

If you are already knowledgeable about alternative

healing and alternative medicine, you will enjoy the fact that this book is written on multiple levels. Below the surface you will find many nuances that will enable you to immediately increase the effectiveness of your work. For example, the Four Phases of Visionary Quantum Healing, the core method, are fully illustrated in Chapter Four. In Chapter Six, there are additional easy-to-learn techniques for specific maladies, such as headaches and fertility problems, information about how to perform distance healing, and more.

The Complete Guide to Visionary Quantum Healing is a pragmatic book. It provides the reader with a compendium of theories and techniques – all you need to begin experimenting with and practicing VQH, a non-invasive scientific process. As a non-medical method, it is completely compatible with and complements conventional medical treatment. The success of VQH is not dependent on either the practitioner or the patient having any kind of particular belief system. By not requiring the client to disrobe, VQH promotes the client's comfort and dignity.

Many physical and emotional cases that are challenging, or even impossible, for conventional medicine to treat are cured with a high rate of success using the VQH process.

Finally, as stated in Chapter One, the scientific community has recently discovered that the mind-body connection is real. It is found in the theory of quantum physics. When people finally realize that the doorway to the mind-body connection is all around us and within us, Visionary Quantum Healing will be recognized for its power to heal both mind and body. You can start the realization now by reading this book.

In Light,

Mike Doty

Table of Contents

Publisher's Note 2

Dedication 3

Acknowledgments 4

Foreword 6

Introduction 20

Chapter One:

The Scientific Basis *24*

Scientific Foundations: 21st-Century Healing 24

A Basis in Quantum Physics 29

Applications to Healing 31

Theoretical Foundations of Visionary Quantum Healing 35

The Vibrational Healing Approach 36

Non-Vibrational Healing Approaches 38

Genesis and Light 41

Laser: Light as a Healing Principle 43

The Life Force of the Body: Creation of the Energy Field 47

Chapter Two: The Concepts 59

The Uses of Negativity and Its Interlink with Positivity 59

Visionary Quantum Healing 63

The Essence of Visionary Quantum Healing 69

Vibrational versus Visionary Quantum Healing 72

Vision and Visionary Quantum Healing 74

Health: Wholeness versus Foreign Entities 76

Is Visionary Quantum Healing for Me? 80

To Believe or Not to Believe:
That is the Question 82

The Sufferer and the Conscious
Visionary Healer 84

Chapter Three:

Ancient Wisdom *87*

The Chakras and the Secret
Teachings of All Ages 87

The Seven Primary Western Chakras 90

The Seven Major Hindu Chakras 92

Therapeutic Transformation for Healing 94

A Friend's Call for Help 96

"Rediscovery is
Every Bit as Good as Discovery" 100

Background for the Four Phases 101

Chapter Four: The Four Phases of Visionary Quantum Healing 119

Phase 1: Relaxation and Feeling
the Depth of Pain 119

Phase 2: Concentration and Establishing
the Healing Energy Link 126

Phase 3: Healing with Pure Natural Air, Light, and Healing Energy 133

Phase 4: Cleansing the Body and the Seven Chakras 139

Aftermath: Protection and Restoring Potency 145

The Qualified Practitioner: Mere Imitation Could Be Deadly 146

Chapter Five: *The History* *149*

A Child's Gift 149

Healing and the Six-Day War 150

Learning from My Own Dreams 153

From the Tehilim (Psalms) of King David 157

The Impact of Rabbi Shimon Bar-Yochaii 163

Chapter Six:
More Healing Methods *168*

Dr. Richard Bloom.
Demonstrates on Salomon Cohn 168

Instant Cure for Janet Parks 181

Natural Light: Healing Energy
Empowerment 186

Awesome Healing Power 189

Healing and Hypno-meditation 191

The Dream of Human Limb Regeneration:
21st-Century Healing 197

Method: Treating Fertility Problems 198

Headache and Pain Elimination 201

Absentee Visionary Quantum Healing Treatment 204

Psychic Coincidences 208

Chapter Seven: A Final Note 211

A Near-Death Experience Occasions Great Discovery 211

Free Fall and Out-of-Body Experience 214

Confirmation of Being Saved By Angels 218

From Agony to Ecstasy: Moments of Discovery 219

The Attentive Angel of Love 221

The Link to Salomon through Past Lives 224

How VQH Differs From Well-known "Medical" Healing Techniques 228

Frequently Asked Questions About Visionary Quantum Healing 235

Conclusion 250

Appendix A: Legal Forms 254

Healing and the Law 254

Client Information 255

Client Agreement and Release from Liability 257

Release and Consent Form 258

Appendix B: White House

Commission Final Report on Health and Alternative Medicine 259

Appendix C:

Case Studies and Testimonials 266

Case Study #1: Healing Other Healers 266

Testimonial #1 268

Case Study #2: Francisco Alessi 271

Testimonial #2 272

Case Study #3: Max Schlesinger 273

Testimonial #3 274

Case Study #4: Sason Gazel 275

Testimonial #4 276

Case Study #5: George Benson 277

Testimonial #5 278

Case Study #6: Mike Doty 279

Testimonial #6 280

Case Study #7: Guy Gardocki 281

Testimonial #7 282

Appendix D *284*

About the Author 284

The Body and Mind Prototype Curative 286

Papa Albert (poem) 288

Bibliography 290

Index 297

Introduction

Visionary Quantum Healing emerges from a cluster of contemporary outlooks. This revolutionary modality of healing is an alternative, non-holistic and non-conventional medical treatment based on scientific concepts and research. It relies on a process of natural air and light energy to restore energy flow and eliminate all unhealthy entities (diseases) within the client's body, mind, and soul. Thus, it addresses the client's physical and emotional condition. It is non-invasive, non-verbal, and requires no touching, so the client need not disrobe. Visionary Quantum Healing successfully treats difficult cases, and most clients need only one treatment. The procedures in this book are easy for practitioners, clients, and students to learn and use.

Unlike other approaches, the VQH system does

not require the client to embrace any belief system, nor is it constricted by one. Belief systems are inherently negative: they are typically built on intolerance for ambiguity and carry implicit, self-destructive threats. The effectiveness of the Ayurvedic healing system and traditional Chinese medicine depend on the client holding certain beliefs about balance and spirit. Though concepts of balance and spirit are useful for diagnosis, Visionary Quantum Healing does not rely on them. Indeed, VQH does not require diagnosis to produce consistently effective treatment when delivered by an expert practitioner. Moreover, its results are immediate.

One might point out that often positive beliefs can contribute to healing. Indeed, even placebo effects can be dramatic. To this observation, I would reply that if a belief system works for you, you have my blessing. I do not use the word "blessing" frivolously, for I personally believe in both VQH and the power of prayer.

I have observed this power in the faith of my ancestors.

The most important point is that holistic and medical approaches are not working for many of us and their effects may not extend beyond immediate relief. The International Classification of Disease or ICD-10 (World Health Organization, 1992-1994) lists about 10,000 diseases and other medical conditions. Only a minority are curable by holistic and conventional methods. While these approaches may offer relief of symptoms, VQH offers an immediate and lasting curative.

This book will serve as a teaching manual for the VQH process. It is enhanced by illustrations that depict the Four-Phase Process with five steps per phase. The book includes extensive scientific research as well as additional curative processes for headache, for various injuries, and for fertility problems. I have included a section on hypno-meditation, absentee healing treatment, and frequently asked questions. Also included are client information forms, release and consent forms, contracts, a section on healing and the law of healing, instructive case studies, professional and client testimonials, the White House Commission Report, a recommended book list, an index, and other useful features.

While *The Complete Guide to Visionary Quantum Healing* will present material that comes from scientific research and religious tradition, the reader should remain mindful that VQH does not derive from any one religion.

I have drawn from Jewish, Hindu and Buddhist teachings, as well as dreams and visions. Contemporary science forms the basis for several key assumptions. Based on the revolutionary Four Phases, Visionary Quantum Healing is the secret to life.

Chapter One The Scientific Basis

1. Scientific Foundations: 21st-Century Healing

21 September 1998

Dear Salomon ,

My daughter Elizabeth was sick for over three weeks with fever every day. She had pains in her wrist. Some days she could not write or use her hands. Some days she needed crutches during this illness, when she had difficulty walking. My husband, who is a physician and I, a nurse, were very worried and very scared during this period. Elizabeth had a healing session with you on a Saturday evening. By Sunday, she was feeling much better and she soon made a full recovery. Today, six months later, she is in excellent health. We believe your healing session was a blessing for Elizabeth and our family.

Sincerely,

Angela G. Amador, Nurse Practitioner

The day I received this letter I decided to go forward with my quest for the scientific foundations of Visionary Quantum Healing.

VQH is based on the key scientific concepts of electromagnetism and quantum physics that emerged during the 19th and 20th centuries and, because of my own background and training, is based to a significant degree on the sacred writings of Jewish Scripture. These concepts challenge ideas that were prevalent during the Age of Reason, which limited notions of mechanism (the fundamental processes involved in or responsible for a natural phenomenon) that had held sway for over two centuries.

One of these scientific ideas is that of unified modes of energy. In 1873, Scottish physicist James Clerk Maxwell published a unified conception of electricity and magnetism as a single force: electromagnetism. Maxwell was much admired by Albert Einstein, who came up with the energy field theory. Einstein's General Theory of Relativity imagined a stretchable fabric of space and time that generates gravity, thereby collapsing the dualities of space and time, matter and energy.

In *Vibrational Medicine: New Choices for Healing Ourselves*, Dr. Richard Gerber writes that "the Einsteinian paradigm as applied to vibrational medicine sees human beings as networks of complex energy fields that interface with physical/cellular systems. Vibrational medicine uses specialized forms of electromagnetic energy to positively affect those energetic systems that may be out of balance due to disease states."[1] Moving beyond vibrational approaches, Visionary Quantum Healing engages the human body's energy field with air and light, and the effects are realized on the physical cellular level. The utilization of natural light in VQH builds upon Einstein's

1. Gerber, Richard, *Vibrational Medicine: New Choices for Healing Ourselves,* Bear & Co. (1988) p. 39

keen interest in the much-debated question of whether light consists of particles or waves.

Another expression of this holistic outlook is the belief, advanced by several scientists and philosophers, that consciousness or spirit is not separate from matter. The past century has heard many scientific calls for such holism. In 1925, in his theory of Process Reality, the famous philosopher Alfred North Whitehead wrote that "Nature is a structure of evolving processes. The reality is the process."[2] Whitehead, a brilliant mathematician, was also fascinated by the natural world. He shifted his focus to biology and came to develop an idea of "nature upon the concept of organism, and not upon the concept of matter."[3] At about the same time, 1928, Sir Arthur Eddington, an astrophysicist famous for his work supporting Einstein's

2. Whitehead, Alfred North, *Science and the Modern World*, The Free Press (1967), p. 72)
3. Ibid, p.75

Theory of Relativity, contended that "the stuff of the world is mind-stuff," and in 1952 prominent quantum physicist Wolfgang Pauli suggested that "Physics and psyche (that is, matter and mind) could be seen as complementary aspects of the same reality."[4]

Despite the implications for medical treatment, Western medicine has been slow to incorporate the implications of holism. Fortunately, some doctors, like Richard Gerber, have broken with the traditional Western notion of the human body as a mechanism: "The unseen connection between the physical body and the subtle forces of spirit holds the key to understanding the inner relationship between matter and energy ...consciousness itself is a kind of energy that is integrally related to the cellular expression of the physical body."[5]

4. Willis, Harman, and Sahtouris, Elisabeth, *Biology Revisioned*, North Atlantic Books (1998), p. 172
5. Gerber, Richard, *Vibrational Medicine: New Choices for Healing Ourselves,* Bear & Co. (1988), p. 44

2. A Basis in Quantum Physics

VQH takes place on the most subtle plane of reality. Contemporary physics, particularly the quantum mechanics pioneered by Erwin Schrödinger, Werner Heisenberg and Niels Bohr, shows that not only is matter a form of energy, but also that matter consists of vibrating particles or charges of energy. To physicist Schrödinger it was clear that the structure of living matter differs from the type of matter his colleagues generally studied. While physicists studied "periodic crystals," biologists were studying "aperiodic crystals," thought to be the building blocks of life. A periodic crystal has a repeating pattern of atoms forming a crystal lattice. An aperiodic crystal exhibits crystalline properties but does not have the repeating pattern of atoms.

According to science writer James Gleick, "The

difference was like the difference between wallpaper and tapestry, between the regular repetition of pattern and the rich, coherent variation of an artist's creation."[6] Gleick goes on to describe Schrödinger's unusual view, that life was both orderly and complex was a truism ; [yet] "to see aperiodicity as the source of its special qualities verged on the mystical."[7]

According to quantum theory, when a solid surface such as a table top or stone is examined under an electron microscope, it appears dynamic, vibrational, and porous. Atoms, the building blocks of our material world, actually consist of far more space than matter. This means that matter, including flesh, has more in common with air, a key element in quantum healing, than might readily be perceived.

6. Gleick, James, *Chaos: Making a New Science*, Viking (1987), p. 299
7. Ibid, p. 300

3. Applications to Healing

Both microscopic and macroscopic space, the subatomic and celestial realms, consist predominantly of open space, leaving relatively great expanses between the nucleus and the electron shell (even between one subatomic particle and the next), although most of us tend to experience existence as a series of material encounters. When we are ill, a friend might ask, "What's the matter? " But matter is only part of the picture. When we are sick, our naturally healthy energy flow in the interatomic spaces is often blocked by foreign entities.

The Visionary Quantum healer tunes into the spaces within and between matter, where light thrives. Intuitively he or she understands the paradox that both modern physics and traditional mysticism have known: that on progressively more subtle levels of experience, "reality" is energy and light. The Visionary Quantum healer treats disease using the four-phase process covered later in the book, to return healthy energy flows to the entire human being.

As quantum theory asserts, no one can be a totally objective observer of reality. On the contrary, our methodology often determines or affects what we perceive. When struck by a beam of light from an electron microscope, electrons behave in atypical ways. The more the investigator blows up a photo image, the more the image becomes distorted.

Acknowledging this "observer effect," Visionary Quantum healers recognize that they must participate in the treatment while they actively engage with and influence the energy flow of the client. They interact on the most subtle human energy field and, through the infusion of "light," are able to heal or make whole. Although these healers do not have to make a diagnosis in order to deliver effective treatment, some opt to do so. Visually scanning the client to create a holographic picture of the client's energy fields, these healers beam and bounce a healing light source on the client. Just as a doctor may first X-ray a client to "see" the client on a deeper level in order to ascertain the problem and determine a possible cure, a Visionary Quantum healer visually scans the body of the client to observe the symptoms as well as the root cause of the condition.

In *Alchemical Studies*, Carl Jung wrote, "We are reminded of the days of creation, of the time when consciousness arose, when the primordial unity of being was barely disturbed by the twilight of reflection, and man swam like a fish in the water."[8] In similarly holistic ways, VQH attempts to see the person as a unified whole, as more than the sum of his or her parts.

8. Jung, Carl, *Alchemical Studies,* Princeton University Press (1967), p. 265

4. Theoretical Foundations Of Visionary Quantum Healing

In this section we will look at the theoretical foundations for several major methods of healing before moving into full explication of the theoretical basis of Visionary Quantum Healing. We will look at vibrational and non-vibrational approaches, including Ayurvedic, homeopathic, and allopathic concepts of healing. Then we will examine the role of light, the creation of energy fields, multidimensional negativity, the importance of air, and the role of consciousness. Finally, we will explore the theoretical and conceptual bases of Visionary Quantum Healing.

5. The Vibrational Healing Approach

Let's begin with the outlooks that are characteristic of vibrational medicine. If someone is blocking a doorway, he or she can be commanded to move or can be physically moved by force. Similarly, disease can be physically removed or can be commanded to leave by the practitioner's summoning a superior authority. In the Indian Vedas, particularly in the Bhagavata Purana, it is observed that the moon reflected on a pool of water appears to quiver with the ripples. The Vedas use the relationship of the moon to the water as an analogy for the relationship between the soul and the body-mind-ego. The soul is eternal, but when it identifies with the transient conditions of the body, mind and ego, it becomes ill because it has falsely identified with an ephemeral and illusory condition. A person is normally aware of his inner body only when he feels sick or in pain. This illusory identification produces "dis-ease," meaning "not at ease." The soul is uncomfortable or ill. Vibrational healing attempts to treat the diseased soul and restore wholeness.

In *Vibrational Medicine*, Dr. Gerber also draws on the concept of wholeness, "the mind/body/spirit complex." Using vibrational medicine, Dr. Gerber "seeks to heal the physical body by integrating and balancing the higher energetic systems which create the physical/cellular patterns of manifestation."[9] He believes that the subtle connection between the body and "the spirit reveals the inner relationship between matter and energy. [Consciousness] is a kind of energy integrally connected

9. Gerber, Richard, *Vibrational Medicine: New Choices for Healing Ourselves,* Bear & Co. (1988), p. 43

to the body. Vibrational medicine attempts to treat people with pure energy."[10] Similarly, the Kabbalistic practice of Tikkun calls for healing based on conceiving matter as energy, and humans as beings of energy. Tikkun means "healing, mending, restoring, fixing, correcting."

6. Non-Vibrational Healing Approaches

Three of the world's great healing traditions do not use a vibrational approach: the Ayurvedic, the homeopathic, and the allopathic. The first is Eastern in origin; the other two are Western.

The traditional Ayurvedic system of medicine is based on the ancient customs, beliefs, and practices of the Hindu culture. In Sanskrit, *ayur* means "life" and *veda* means "knowledge"; thus, Ayurveda has come to mean "the

10. Gerber, Richard, *Vibrational Medicine: New Choices for Healing Ourselves*, Bear & Co. (1988), p. 44

science of life." Ayurveda is the science of self-healing. Its practitioners consider the human body a great source of knowledge and urge clients to take responsibility for their own healing.

Ayurveda pays close attention to balance in the person's life. Balance is the natural order, while imbalance is disorder. Health is order, disease is disorder. Moreover, energy is required for the body to function. Ayurveda, which views the cause of disease as a lack of proper cellular function due to an excess or deficiency of one kind of energy, treats disease with combinations of ingested herbs, purgatives, and rubbing oils.

The second great healing tradition is homeopathy. The word "homeopathy" derives from the Greek *homeo*, "like" and *pathy*, "disease". Homeopathy is a system that follows the "law of similars," in which the treatment produces symptoms similar to those of the illness. Homeopathy treats disease with minute doses of remedies that would ordinarily, in healthy persons, produce the symptoms of the disease. Popular in Europe, homeopathy employs the full spectrum of natural substances to dissipate the toxicities of an illness. The crystalline network of the human body assists in transducing and distributing subtle energies of homeopathic remedies to their appropriate paths of action.

The third healing system is allopathic. The word "allopathic" comes from the Greek *allos*, "other" and *pathy*, "disease." It treats disease by "other" or "dissimilar" means. Allopathy refers to all Western medical approaches not based on homeopathic assumptions, including the essential separation of mind and body and the belief that the body is basically a chemical mechanism, an incredible machine. Western medicine relies on surgery and pharmaceuticals to provide broad-spectrum relief and includes essentially technological approaches to the treatment of illness.

7. Genesis and Light

From the beginning of creation up to the present cutting edge of scientific technology, light has occupied the premier position among all phenomena. In science, light exhibits properties as both a particle and a wave, embodied in the massless and chargeless photon traveling as a quantum of electromagnetic energy that has momentum.

In the book of Genesis, God said, "Let there

be light" (Gen. 1.3). But a few verses later, God also pronounced that there are "two great lights; the greater light to rule the day, and the lesser light to rule the night" (Gen.1.16). Genesis is a book about divisions, but the divisions are not always absolute.

Light is also important in modern science. Einstein's famous formula for total mass-energy conversion, $E=mc^2$, is based on his insight that energy and mass are inter-related with the speed of light.

Much of modern scientific equipment is based on laser-technology. From CD players to advanced laser medical technologies, light is the most powerful and safest means for many ends. In VQH, air and light perform their work on the most primal and subtle level. Light can also work at a distance, because it travels freely through space.

8. Laser: Light as a Healing Principle

"Laser" means "light amplification by stimulated emission of radiation." In a device that emits laser light, the majority of the atoms or molecules have been converted to an excited energy state. This allows the device to emit coherent light of a precise wavelength in an intense narrow beam. With this technology, diseases once deemed "incurable" are now routinely cured. The miraculous becomes mundane. A miracle is an event that apparently contradicts known scientific laws and is hence thought to be the result of supernatural causes. The word "miracle" derives from *miraculum*, Latin, "a strange thing" and *mirari,* French, "to wonder at." But there is nothing supernatural about Visionary Quantum Healing.

Lasers are essential to holograms, three-dimensional images created by an interference pattern of two interacting laser beams. The Holographic Principle states that holograms are unique and that they represent an energy interference pattern in which every piece of the hologram contains the information of the whole. Physicist David Bohm, Professor of Theoretical Physics at Birkbeck College of the University of London, based his theory of energy on the hologram. The Holographic Principle is used in VQH. Indeed, the healer can reconstruct the client's entire energy system by working with his or her holographic aura. The shade, shape, and texture of the aura will indicate the kind of disease or imbalance that is present.

Repeatedly, people are astounded at how they

are healed by a Visionary Quantum healer without being touched. The answer is simple. It is not possible to touch a person's holographic energy fields with human hands. However, the light emanating from the Visionary Quantum healer's laser-like vision rapidly bounces back and forth over the client's body like a stream of fire and permeates the client's entire energy system, purging disease and imbalance through the crown chakra at the top of the head (the chakras are more fully discussed in Chapter 3). Air and light energy encounter no barriers. The pulsing movement of their energy facilitates the complete restoration of the client's healthy aura.

VQH is not complicated. Clients, students, and health practitioners may rapidly become properly qualified to handle this method of high-voltage energy healing. The purpose of this book is to explain the VQH process to ordinary people and potential clients, and to be a teaching manual for those wanting to become practitioners. The subtleties of being a Visionary Quantum healer can be learned by studying this book and by attending my teaching seminar, or by learning the process from another experienced practitioner. More information on the seminars is at my web site, www.drcohn.net.

9. The Life Force of the Body: Creation of the Energy Field

Much as lasers may be blocked, so too the body may experience energy blockages caused by abnormal functions in one or more chakras. Energy blockage refers to an interruption of the flow of energy through the body's energy system. Deborah Cowens, in *A Gift for Healing*, writes, "Our ancestors taught that the physical body is the creation of the energetic field, which itself is part of the larger spiritual world."[11] In the same way, health, as well as most forms of illness, begin in the energy field and ultimately manifest in the physical body.

According to Cowens, "The physical manifestation of disease is the last stop in the process that began in the

11. Cowens, Deborah, *A Gift for Healing,* Crown Trade Paperbacks (1996) p.82

Photograph of Dr. Cohn's Psychic Aura

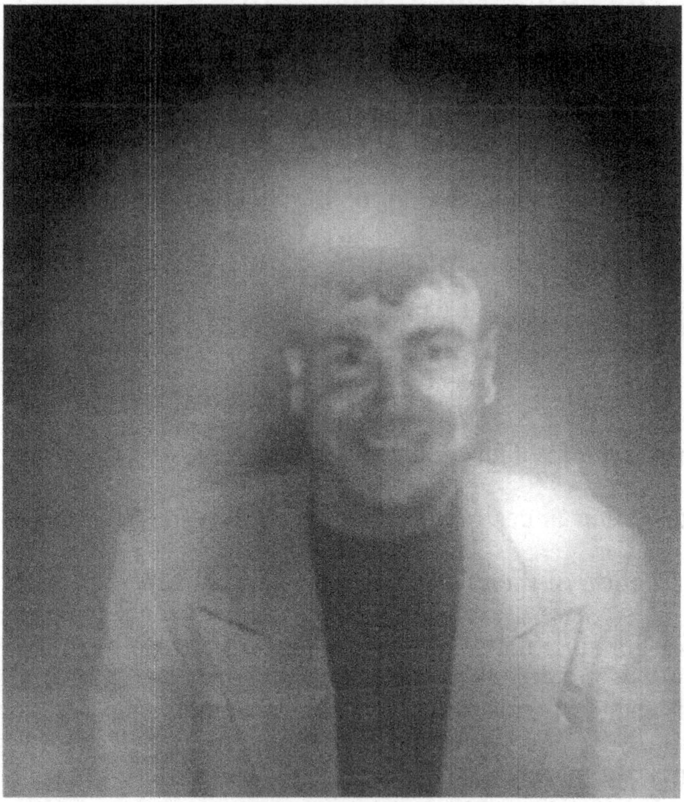

This photograph of Dr. Cohn's psychic aura, taken with a high density Polaroid camera at the American Board of Hypnotherapy Convention 2000, is a view of the human aura. With some effort and recommended reading (see page 59) the reader can learn to see the aura as well.

energetic field. Whenever a blockage manifests in the field, life energy is prevented from flowing optimally to the body or to a specific place within the body. When numerous blockages manifest, the flow of the life force is diminished. As I have said, without life force the body cannot survive. Without optimal life force, the body cannot sustain health."[12]

This idea of a life force has ancient roots. The ancient Taoist concept of Ch'i is expressed in Chinese medicine as the energy of the body, which may be blocked if the person is diseased. Life force has also appeared in the writings of the "Righteous" Rabbi Shimon Bar-Yochaii, an author of the Kabbalah in the second century, in the writings of Moses Maimonides, doctor and foremost Jewish philosopher of the twelfth century, in the thinking

12. Cowens, Deborah, *A Gift for Healing*, Crown Trade Paperbacks (1996) p. 82

of the modern philosopher Henri Bergson, and in work of the 20th century novelist D. H. Lawrence. Like many of his contemporaries, Lawrence was interested in occult symbolism and theosophy as a source of primitive theology. He expressed the life force in the metaphors of spirit and the supernatural.

Far too often, however, the Western approach neglects the body's energy flow. The root cause of disease is eclipsed by an emphasis on alleviating the external symptoms. People do not want to hear that their behavior, diet, or lifestyle may have to be modified. In the language of advertising, they want immediate relief.

On the other hand, many holistic methods require such dramatic behavioral changes that most people find it impossible to implement them all, or to maintain the strict standards necessary for the method to take full effect. While delivering immediate relief, VQH requires no conscious effort by the client. The power to heal lies within the practitioner and his or her ability to create the transfer of the healing potential of air and light energy to the client.

In addition to producing heat, gases and energy, every form of life emits an aura consisting of a glow of color around the body. This aura reveals health, mood and thoughts. The concept of auras has been around throughout recorded history.

The challenge in recent years has been to find a way of recording auras in an objective manner. Recording and viewing auras in a scientific, repeatable manner may lead to their use in the diagnosis and healing of health, psychological and emotional problems.

Historically, knowledge of auras comes from the psychics who can see them. They say that the color of an individual's aura, and the distance it radiates from a body, provides information about the health of the person. The hue and intensity of the aura are said to fluctuate constantly as the individual changes moods, thoughts and levels of fatigue. A widely agreed catalogue of aura qualities has been developed, along with an understanding of what they mean. For example, a green aura reflects intellectual factors, while any brown or gray shades reflect disease. However, science has not gathered any definitive results, and different techniques in photography are constantly being evolved to try to capture auras on a solid substance.

The first person to use auras for medical purposes was Walter Kilner, the head of the electro-therapy department at St. Thomas Hospital in London in 1911. Kilner discovered that by looking through colored glass he could see an outline of light surrounding the patient's body. He noticed that the light changed shape, intensity and color as the patient's health altered. Kilner was the only one who could see the light, and it was not until 1939 that his discoveries were taken any further.

Semyon Kirlian, a Russian hospital electrician, stumbled by chance upon a completely unique method of photography. By placing a living object on a photographic plate and running a high voltage through it, the most amazing image of strange colors appeared as a halo around the subject. Kirlian and his wife, Valentina, perfected the technique. The first photograph they took showed a leaf with millions of orange and turquoise light dots seemingly emanating from the leaf's veins, and a bizarre aura around the leaf edges. Over time they conducted many experiments and even developed an instrument that would show auras in motion. They noted that healthy, vital subjects created pictures with the most distinct, radiant outlines while withered and dying subjects would result in very weak auras. Kirlian also proposed and demonstrated the theory that different colors emanated with different moods, feelings and thoughts.

Starting around 1970, Thelma Moss, a parapsychologist at the University of California, became convinced in the power of auras for medical purposes. She promoted the view that Kirlian's discovery was a way of showing bioenergy as a tangible, provable subject. Moss visited the Soviet Union to discuss techniques with paranormal researchers there. She wanted to use Kirlian auras as a diagnostic tool, and believed the subject represented the next major step forward for the medical establishment.

In 1975, Gary K. Poock, Professor of Operations Research and Man-Machine Systems at the U.S. Navy Postgraduate School at Monterey, California, developed a bioelectrographic motion picture method using a light intensifier for improving brightness. This system reveals the dramatic dynamics of the discharge process which are invisible at the long exposure times of still photography. In 1976, Poock made a first step to the quantification of the electrographic picture by introducing an image-analytic technique. A paradigmatic investigation of electrography, published in 1976 and 1978 and partly sponsored by the U.S. Department of Defense, was conducted for 6 years by a multidisciplinary team headed by William Eidson, Professor of Physics at Drexel University, Philadelphia (Pehek et al., 1976; Eidson et al., 1978). Among other things, the study points to the typical instability of the equipment used in most investigations and the wide range of parameters that have to be controlled for the successful operation of the method. It also gives recommendations for optimum discharge technology and recordings systems, such as transparent electrodes and image-intensified film or video recording systems which allow for contactless image recording without interference between the specimen/ electrode circuit and the recording medium, and the use of image analysis and the spectral analysis of the discharge process. The study concluded that electrography was able to image electrical parameters of a specimen in real time, making it a possible field mapping tool for the energy fields surrounding living organisms which possibly were able to modulate "space impedance". The important task of carefully analyzing all of the parameters influencing the bioelectrographic image which the Drexel team had started and many since then have called for, was undertaken by Mark de Payrebrune, then graduate student of Electrical Engineering at McGill University at Montreal, Canada, for his master's thesis in 1984 (de Payrebrune, 1984).

To connect with the aura, focus on the region of the third eye between the eyebrows. After a few moments, you will begin to feel and see colors floating and filling you. Go with the feeling and imagine how the colors are encircling you. Use your imagination to create a huge bubble, preferably green (the most peaceful color) and float inside it. Stay like this for about 10 minutes.

To increase the sense of general well-being, use aromatic oils known to have a calming effect on the nervous system. About eight drops in warm water in a glass half full. Bergamot oil diminishes anxiety and nervousness; sandalwood for tranquility and serenity; lavender for peace; orange (or any citrus) contributes to a better frame of mind; ti bar, an Indian mixture which increases serenity; cedar and frankincense for focus and for inner peace. to identify and align one's personal frequency (Aura) to a more balanced internal electromagnetic field.

We all have a demonstrable life force surrounding us. It is only a matter of time before some unquestionable technique is devised, and a whole new world of personal care is unveiled.

Kirlian Photography–Salomon's Hands of Fire

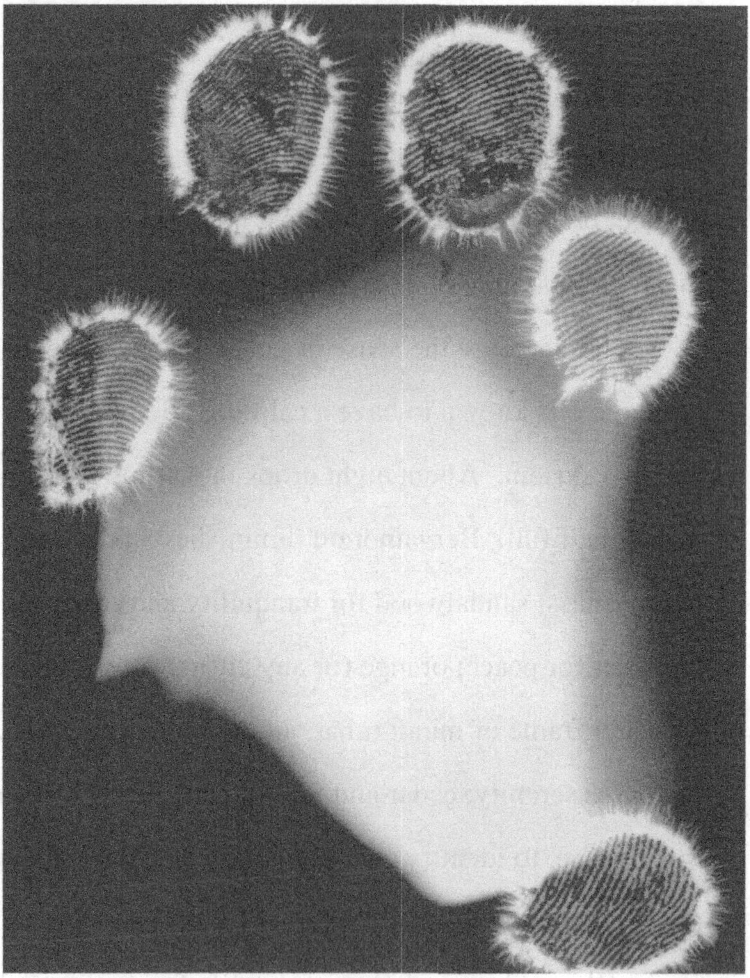

This remarkable image of Salomon Cohn's hand was taken with Kirlian photography, which uses high voltage to show the bio energy or aura flowing from an object. We all have bio energy that can be increased in intensity for use in the Visionary Quantum Healing process. By rubbing your hands and concentrating, you will be able to increase the energy from the palm of your hand..

Chapter Two *The Concepts*

10. The Uses of Negativity and Its Interlink with Positivity

Not only is the unimpeded flow of energy important, it is also crucial to acknowledge the positive and negative charges of the body's energy. Modern psychotherapy and self-help methods have placed much emphasis on exploring the unexplored, espousing the power of positive thinking, self-affirmation, and creative visualization. They have helped many people to find direction in their lives and realize their aspirations. But, the value of the negative has been overlooked; the negative remains relatively unexplored.

I am not promoting negativity in its ordinary sense of self-deprecation, low self-esteem, or any self-defeating, self-depleting waste of human energy and potential. It is well known that a toxic mind sometimes leads to a toxic body. However, the power of spiritual negativity in many areas, especially as a healing resource, is virtually unlimited—with powerful positive effects as the outcome. Any type of thorough therapeutic process attempts to reverse the conditions of disease, generating a positive healthy complement.

Sometimes even the darkest moments can lead to remarkable positives.

My early rearing and education were in Israel. When I was fourteen, I joined a kibbutz as a continuation of my high school studies. It was required that all members of the commune learn to garden and farm, so I learned to cultivate grapes and grapefruit, and how to care for horses and milk cows. The communal lifestyle intrigued me.

One day I observed far off in the distance an elderly man limping toward me, carrying a wooden box. I approached him, offering my help. Thankful, he handed me the box. He had been invited by the kibbutz to photograph and document its various activities.

As we walked in the summer heat, the man rolled up his sleeves, revealing an identification number tattooed on his arm by the Nazis. I asked probing questions. During the war, he told me, he fought against the Germans in Warsaw, Poland. He lived and fought as a partisan, both to keep his dignity as a Jew and to express compassion for his fellow man. He was shot by an SS German officer, and took a bullet in his hip. After his capture he was sent to a Nazi concentration camp, then transferred to another at Auschwitz to be gassed and cremated. As his time neared, the camp was suddenly liberated by Russian Red Army forces. He implored me to never forget our Jewish brothers and sisters who died in the Holocaust, to learn the history of the Jewish people, and to teach it to my children and grandchildren.

Then I asked him about photography. His eyes widened, sparkling, as he spoke of the joys and magic of photography: from the negative a positive picture evolves. I was enchanted by this process and after I moved to New York in 1968, I actually owned and operated camera stores. Over time, this knowledge of photography helped me better understand the process of VQH and its reversal of illness.

With the VQH system, the better the negativity, the better the balancing with the positivity. It is a system built upon reversal.

It is not necessary for a client undergoing VQH to understand how this method works for it to be effective, but for practitioners attempting to become skilled in VQH and for training others, understanding it is absolutely essential.

11. Visionary Quantum Healing

How does a Visionary Quantum practitioner differ from vibrational, Ayurvedic, homeopathic, and allopathic healers? While the other healers rely on beliefs, on mind and spirit, or on chemical concepts, the Visionary Quantum healer works with a Four-Phase Process that uses air and light energy.

To the Visionary Quantum healer, "vision" means actually seeing reality. I don't know if I developed this gift of X-ray vision or if I was born with the ability to see through the physical being, even when clothed. On a good day I have great accuracy and success. And then I visually scan the client and create a holographic picture of his or her energy fields. When I relax, I can detect breaks in the aura as well as disease entities. A successful VQH treatment gloriously refreshes the aura, making it beautiful, robust, and unbroken. With some focus, effort, and practice using the exercises described later in this book, anyone can see through a human being and determine whether an aura has health and wholeness or if it is full of foreign entities. In *Concerning The Scientific Study Of The Human Aura,* Charles T. Tart describes the science and study of the aura. "What I have tried to do here is to indicate some of the methodological and logical complexities in the field we have been discussing and to point out the need for distinguishing these things, as well as to suggest some methods we can begin to use to get at these phenomena."[13]

13. Tart, Charles T., *Concerning The Scientific Study Of The Human Aura,* Journal of the Society for Psychical Research (1972)

12. The Essence of Visionary Quantum Healing

A. Healing with Air

Because air is necessary for life, it is also necessary for health and healing. Air is literally vital, for in many languages the word for "air" implies a vital presence and often actually means "life." To understand the theoretical basis of VQH, we will start with the etymologies of the words for air in two ancient languages, Greek and Hebrew. In early Greek, the language of the poet Homer, *psyche* meant "the breath of life," and only later came to mean "mind" and "soul." Similarly, in ancient Hebrew, the word *ruach* meant not only "air" but also "life," "force," "oxygen," "spirit," "wind," and "healing force." VQH incorporates life force as it heals by making use of air.

While the exact means by which air, particularly moving air, is able to heal remains unknown, its effects have been noted among the survivors of the atomic bomb that was dropped during World War II at Nagasaki, Japan, on August 9, 1945. Those who continued living near the ocean exhibited greater rates of survival. This higher rate, it seems quite possible, was due to the moving air of relatively pollution-free sea breezes. Gently pulsing air, whether from a breeze or another source of air movement, has salutary effects. It relaxes a person and encourages the life force within him or her. Clean air clears pollutants from both living tissue and the environment.

Anyone can test the healing force of the wind from the ocean by standing for half an hour by the seashore. You will feel as tired as if you had been working hard nonstop for several hours, and yet this feeling of having participated in physical exertion will be accompanied by an overall sense of cleansing and healing.

In VQH, the method is to rapidly bounce air back and forth on the surface of the body, much like a bobbing balloon. This creates an alternation of slightly higher and lower pressures over the surface of the body, something which naturally occurs only during rapid breathing. The importance of air as a component of life is discussed in detail in the next chapter, where the relationship between air and soul is discussed. In my experience, the healing process has been much more successful when air is combined with natural light and bodily energy, or life force, by a trained practitioner.

B. Healing with Natural Light Energy

In *Vibrational Medicine,* Dr. Gerber explains, "From the simple cobalt machine to the linear accelerator, new ways of delivering therapeutic doses of energy to the body have become more and more sophisticated."[14]

From this perspective on energy we learn that as modern science has progressed, it has sought subtler and more precise ways of approaching sickness and delivering treatment. So it is only natural, in the evolution of healing processes, to move further away from ignorance (darkness) and begin to approach knowledge (light). Visionary Quantum Healing uses natural air and light energy to achieve this goal.

Doctors, geneticists, microbiologists, and

14. Gerber, Richard, M.D., *Vibrational Medicine: New Choices for Healing Ourselves,* Bear & Co. (1988), p. 92

astronomers are always seeking alternative ways of increasing clarity and expanding their range of vision. Continually improving techniques and instrumentation have led to a progressive refinement of scientific knowledge over the centuries, with a corresponding revision of scientific theory. Some casualties along the way have included the replacement of the earth with the sun as the center of the solar system, the phlogiston theory of combustion and the ether theory of light travel. Other theories have been revised, like the addition of the Lorentz Transform to Newtonian mechanics to make it consistent with Einstein's Theory of Special Relativity, $E = \frac{mc^2}{\sqrt{(1-v^2/c^2)}}$. We have learned that when something is seen fully, a more accurate diagnosis can be made and more appropriate treatment given.

Unfortunately, some methods of viewing and treating the inner structure, or the even more subtle cellular level, of the human body may have undesirable side effects. Radiation, chemotherapy, and other treatments have severe side effects, even when they are "effective." Visionary Quantum Healing is extremely sophisticated and totally non-invasive, has no harmful side effects, is one hundred percent safe, and produces lasting results.

A Visionary Healer is not intrusive in any way — he or she does not even touch his client while delivering a full dose of healing natural air and light energy! Natural light has the full spectrum of electromagnetic frequencies derived from the energy processes of the universe, while artificial light is limited in spectrum and does not partake of the natural energy flow.

13. Vibrational vs. Visionary Quantum Healing

Blindness is always a problem. The Hindus tell the famous tale of "The Six Blind Men and the Elephant." This tale is a parable of subjectivity. What each man perceives as an elephant depends on where he touches the elephant, i.e., the trunk, the ears, a leg, a tusk, and so on.

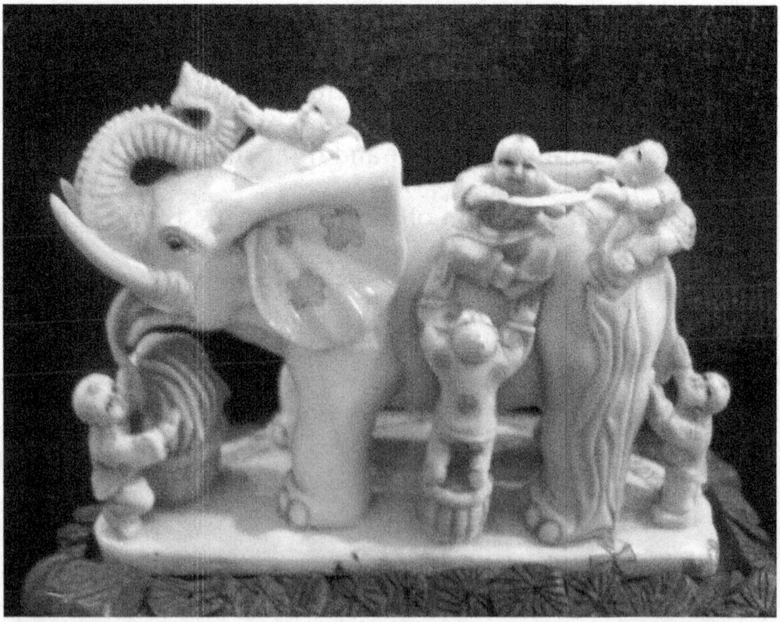

The Sufis, who are Muslim mystics, tell the story of a blind man who was riding a horse and dropped his riding crop. He got down from his horse, mistakenly grabbed a sleeping cobra, and then remounted. An old man nearby warned the blind man that he had picked up a poisonous snake, but the blind man ignored him. After a while, the blind man began to whip his horse with the sleeping cobra, which abruptly awoke and angrily bit him, killing him with poisonous venom.

The moral is that we have to take guidance from those whose eyes are truly open.

A Visionary Quantum healer is one whose spiritual healing eyes are wide open.

In *Vibrational Medicine,* Dr. Gerber rightly emphasizes the importance of energy flow. Stressing the "unseen connection" between the energies of the body and spirit, he also conceives of consciousness as a form of energy and asserts that vibrational medicine "treats people with pure energy" (pp. 43-44). But Dr. Gerber puts undue emphasis on projecting energy through consciousness. While a Visionary Quantum healer may project energy through consciousness, he or she primarily treats clients with a combination of natural air and light energy.

14. Vision and Visionary Quantum Healing

We have said that vision is one of the essentials of VQH and is necessary for true healing and development. Those great souls who have given society direction spiritually, politically, and otherwise are known as prophets, poets, and great thinkers or, more generally, as visionaries. It is by their vision that human civilization is able to make giant leaps forward.

Without such vision, the body, no matter how strong and healthy, is in constant danger. Western medical doctors can examine or "see" a client with a microscope, an EKG (electrocardiogram), a CAT scan (computed axial tomography X-ray technique that makes a three-dimensional image of the body) and an MRI (magnetic resonance imaging, which can be used to study thin cross-sections of the body). Thus, an entire world not visible to the human eye is revealed. By contrast, a visionary healer may rely on psychic vision in addition to the VQH approach. In either case, it is clear that the most fundamental level of disease is invisible to the eye, making it difficult to identify. Moreover, by drawing on emotional perception, the visionary healer empathizes with human suffering, seeing the client's total health potential.

15. Health: Wholeness versus Foreign Entities

Vision, one of the five physical senses, refers to more than eyesight. Vision also concerns the ability to "see" beyond the surface into the soul or to perceive foreign entities that are inhabiting the physical body. To increase their effectiveness, healers are often acutely sensitive in visual and visionary perception. They may "see" with their hearts and intuition as well as with their eyes. And, they may have a vision of the client's potential wholeness and wellness, identifying intimately with the client on several levels. In one instance, when I was scanning a client's organs, I saw a pulsing from his spleen (see case study of Rimon Issac, pp. 248-252).

This vision may be developed by first shining a

flashlight behind one's finger and observing the visible variations in tissue mass. Note the deeper red under the fingernail compared to the surrounding skin. Follow this by looking at the sun through closed eyelids. Observe the translucent red tissue, similar in appearance to the glow of the finger illuminated by the flashlight. Most likely, dark spots will be seen within the red of the eyelids, similar in appearance to the red under the fingernail in the previous exercise. With continued exposure, the darker red areas will dissolve, leaving a uniform red tone. The darker areas represent disease entities dissipating under the healing gaze. By repeating this exercise, the healer is soon able to see through the fully clothed human body in a similar manner, with locations of disease entities appearing as darkened masses. Learning this technique enables the healer to concentrate on those areas needing the most attention.

"Healing" in its truest sense means "restoring wholeness." Not realizing our potential, we are not complete or whole. This happens when we neglect ourselves or fail to face reality.

Disease, however, does not involve incompleteness; rather, it involves excessive completeness. In engineering, too many dimensions in a drawing over-constrains the design, resulting in confusion to the machinist who makes the part, as to which dimensions have priority. So is it in human completeness. Disease disrupts wholeness and stagnates the person's energy. A Visionary Quantum healer releases this stagnant energy, using his or her own energy as a catalyst to restore healthy energy flow. The energy transfer takes place through the person's chakras. This restoration of healthful natural air and light energy flow will mark the end of pain. Just as clouds sometimes obscure the sun, disease clouds the normal condition of the self. As a result, one loses radiance.

VQH not only restores the normal, healthy condition of the body and soul, but augments the conditions necessary for achieving wholeness or potential. A piece of wood can either be used for firewood, or for a pencil, to write a sonnet. We can lead our lives at a biological level, or we can experience the joys of health and wholeness, celebrating our full physical, emotional, intellectual, and spiritual being.

16. Is Visionary Quantum Healing for Me?

Dr. Richard Gerber has written convincingly about the "shift from Newtonian pharmacokinetic" based medicine toward "Einsteinian pure energetic healing." According to Gerber, "in the New Age that is nearly upon us, the healer/physician will begin to comprehend that the human organism is a series of interacting multidimensional energy fields."[15] Energy-based healing will boost medicine into a higher realm of understanding human suffering and its relief. Gerber's approach relies on beliefs about the nature of energy and consciousness.

Dr. Deepak Chopra also relies on belief systems for his healing approach. In *Quantum Healing*, he says: "Life is a field of unlimited possibilities. Such is the glory

15. Gerber, Richard, M.D., *Vibrational Medicine: New Choices for Healing Ourselves,* Bear & Co. (1988), p. 91

of total flexibility in the human nervous system. This is a tremendously important point. It says we can bypass the limited, bounded choices that we are used to making and go directly to the solution of any problem."[16] His approach is based on belief in choice and unlimited possibilities.

Bypassing the usual limitations, VQH attacks the problem directly, does not work solely from holistic assumptions, and avoids the fallacies of Western and Eastern dualisms such as the mind/matter split.

Using the techniques described in *The Complete Guide to Visionary Quantum Healing*, your healing success will be much more consistent and much more predictable. Your effectiveness in working with others to achieve optimal results will be dramatically increased. You will be able to generate empowering emotional states

16. Chopra, Deepak, *Quantum Healing: Exploring the Frontiers of Mind & Body Medicine*, Bantam Books (1990), p. 228

within yourself, eliminate negative emotions and limiting decisions, identify and change limiting beliefs, and inspire yourself with a compelling future that will have a much better chance of coming true.

17. To Believe or Not Believe: That is the Question

People often ask, "What is your belief system?" In fact, one of my dearest friends, a Ph.D. and healer whose specialty is hypnosomatic therapy, once told me that he would teach me a method of reverse psychology to take the sufferer out of his symptoms just prior to healing. His method teaches the client a psychological belief system. He concluded, "Salomon — you must give them a belief system."

He recalled a client he had attempted to treat by applying what he could observe of my healing methods. He thought he had healed her, but she did not seem mentally stable and was upset with him.

This was terribly alarming to me. "Since when are you treating people using Visionary Quantum Healing? Treating mental cases such as this is potentially dangerous. I have taught you many things—but not everything! You must become properly qualified. At least read my book. Get certified like the rest of my students. Come to my seminar." He had tried to imitate my approach without proper training.

Since he didn't speak to me for a few weeks, I guessed he didn't like my angry response. Three weeks later he did apologize, and said he looked forward to reading my book and taking the training. Now we are closer than ever. The point is this: while we humans need a belief system or worldview in our lives, we do not need to adopt a specific belief system to be healed. Unlike hypnosis, where the client often experiences difficulty adopting a belief in the method, VQH simply asks the client to relax into the healing process. It is important and useful for the practitioner to understand the perspectives expressed here, but the client need not accept them to be healed.

18. The Sufferer and the Conscious Visionary Healer

Consciousness is the basis of everything. It is

with consciousness that I make this statement and you comprehend it. Consciousness is the awareness of feeling. If a client is temporarily rendered unconscious, he or she experiences no feeling. As the anesthesia wears off and consciousness slowly returns, the client gradually begins to feel again.

While the root cause of all suffering is located in the subconscious mind, this cause manifests in the conscious mind. When foreign entities (diseases) enter the body, they first move into the subconscious mind, then the conscious mind.

There is a conscious sufferer, but there is also a conscious healer. VQH takes place on the plane of consciousness and does not work with the unconscious. Totally non-invasive, this method sends energy into the inner being of the suffering person. In order to do this, healers must access not only the diseased life-force energy bodies of clients, but also their own life-force energy. From long and extensive experience they are able to transcend both the physical plane and their own selves. They are able to expand their consciousness so that they are quite literally working on an energetic level that expands to "touch" the diseased energy bodies of the client.

Many clients have stated that during a session they felt an extra pair of hands being placed on them, were surrounded by a glorious light, sometimes with halos, and presented with the gift of Visionary Quantum Healing.

In this chapter we have seen how VQH contrasts with other approaches to healing. VQH relies on natural air and light energy. In the next chapter, we will examine how this amazing alternative can be applied more specifically.

Chapter Three: *Ancient Wisdom*

19. The Chakras and the Secret Teachings of All Ages

Although the chakras are often associated with the Hinduism of the East, they also appear in Western culture. In fact the chakras are nearly universal. For example, the energy centers that appear on the Kabbalistic Tree of Life from the 1st century A.D. roughly correspond to the chakras. According to Kabbalistic scholar Manly Hall, "In this single tree were condensed all the arcana previously scattered throughout the voluminous archives of Kabbalistic literature" (The Secret Teachings of All Ages, p. CXXIII).

The chakras are reflected in the Christian Sacraments: baptism, meaning "All is One"; communion, meaning "Honor One Another"; confirmation, meaning "Honor One's Self"; marriage, meaning "Love is Divine Power"; confession, meaning "Surrender Personal Will to Divine Will"; ordination, meaning "Seek Only the Truth"; and extreme unction, meaning "Live in the Present Moment." They are all related to the *Sefirot*, the paths of the Tree of Life.

Cohn - Visionary Quantum Healing™

Paths Of Wisdom On the Sefirot, the Hebrew The Tree Of Life

Highest Crown Chakra

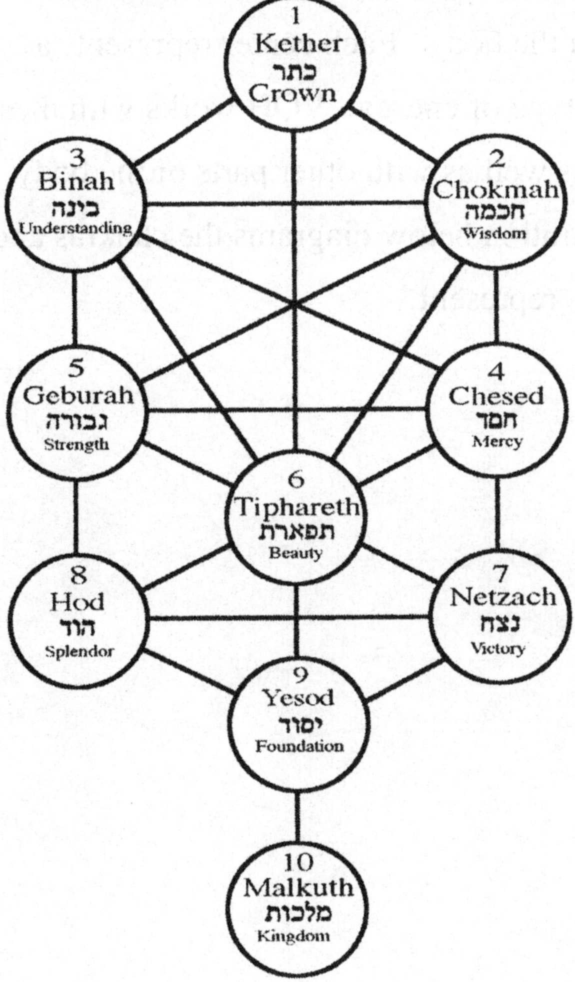

20. The Seven Primary Western Chakras

Chakras are the seven primary energy centers in the body. Each center represents a different type of energy. VQH works with these centers, as well as with other parts of the body. The illustration below diagrams the chakras and what they represent.

The Seven Primary Western Chakras

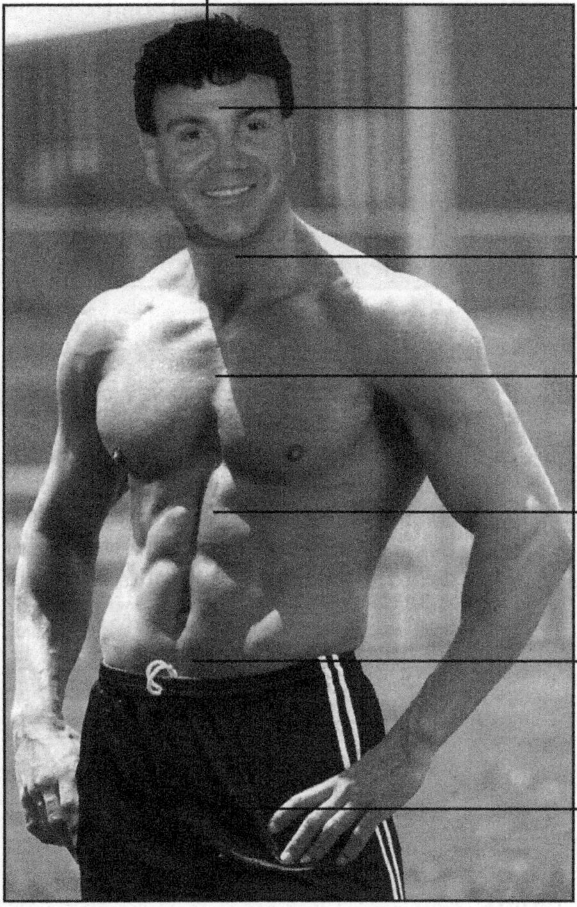

7th Crown Chakra
Pituitary Gland
Spiritual Energy

6th Chakra - Third Eye
Pineal Gland - Psychic/
Perception/Creativity

5th Chakra - Thyroid
Communication Energy

4th Chakra - Heart
Unconditional Love and
Affinity Energy

3rd Chakra -
Just Above the Navel -
Will Power

2nd Chakra -
Ovaries/Testes
Emotional/Sexual Energy

1st Chakra
Base of Spine
Survival Energy

21. The Seven Major Hindu Chakras

In contrast to the Westernized energy centers, the original chakras come from a deeper Hindu tradition discussed in the sutras of Patanjali, who lived in Northern India around 3000 B.C.E. The major chakras include:

1. Sahasrara (crown of the head)
2. Ajna (third eye)
3. Visuddha (throat)
4. Anahata (heart)
5. Manipura (belly)
6. Svadisthana (genital region)
7. Muladhara (seat of the anus)

Beyond these, there are other minor chakras:

a. Surya (the sympathetic nervous system)
b. Chandra (the parasympathetic nervous system)
c. Manas (the mind)

Patanjali's Yoga Sutras

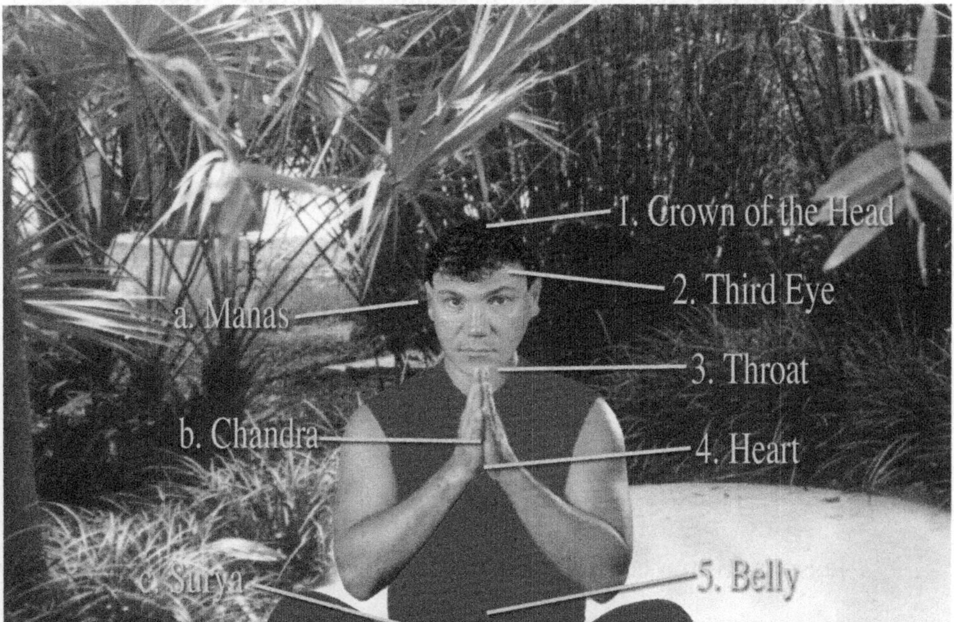

22. Therapeutic Transformation for Healing

There is no room for chronic injury or sickness in a healthy biological organ or human organism. Arrested or blocked life energy flow is the ultimate source of such health problems. Using the Four Phases illustrated in Chapter 4, the Visionary Quantum healer releases stagnant energy, using natural air and light energy, along with his or her own energy, to catalyze the return to healthy energy flow. This transfer of energy takes place through the person's chakras.

The Visionary Quantum healer takes his or her lessons from a central principle of classical physics. Newton's Third Law of Motion states that for every action there is an opposite and equal reaction. Disease is one such reverse action, and it happens in response to a foreign entity. VQH can in turn counter this disease "reaction." But the work of the practitioner would be short-lived if the client returned to stagnant energy.

The key to remaining healthy, disease-free and pain-free is to live in accordance with the healthy energy flow expressed by nature. To this end it is recommended that the client practice a holistic healing modality such as yoga and proper eating. A burst of healthful energy from the Visionary Quantum healer initiates the client's path of awareness. Subsequently, the more clients deepen their awareness, the more they will become conscious of their natural rhythms.

23. A Friend's Call for Help

On May 20, 1998 I received an urgent call from a Latin American friend who lives in Miami. Juan's voice was filled with anxiety and despair.

"Salomon, my sister Vanessa is dying of cancer at a hospital in San Francisco. The doctors say it's hopeless, they can do nothing. Investigative surgery revealed cancer of the liver beyond treatment. She is going to die. I'm flying into San Francisco tomorrow morning. Salomon — I'm begging you to see her. Please, heal my sister!"

His pleading overwhelmed me, and I agreed to treat Vanessa.

Juan's brother Alejandro and sister in-law May-Lee, live in San Francisco. May-Lee, who grew up in Beijing, is a student of holistic medicine. They picked me up at my home the same morning that Juan called, and we drove to the hospital where their sister lay dying. As we drove, the conversation wandered in and out of three languages — English, Spanish, and Chinese. After some small talk, May-Lee asked me a serious question that, although simple on the surface, was profound.

"Salomon — when did healing begin?"

"Healing began with life itself," I answered. "Since the beginning of time, when hurt animals licked their wounds, applying saliva and heat to begin the healing process, and when humans applied saliva from their mouths and heat energy from the palms of their hands to their wounds."

May-Lee was stunned.

"I never heard of such a thing. I have been taught that healing began more than four thousand years ago in China." I, too, was stunned.

Then I recalled reading an article in the *New York Times*. Researchers had discovered that human and bat saliva were linked to interferon, a cellular protein produced in response to viral infection that acts to inhibit viral growth. This healing element in saliva could be used as a curative for cancer. The problem was that treatment required massive doses.

I explained the scientific basis for my statement, along with the theoretical foundations of VQH. May-Lee was grateful. "Thank you for revealing the evolution of healing to me. I will definitely be at your next seminar to learn more about Visionary Quantum Healing."

That afternoon, in Vanessa's room at San Ramon

Hospital I performed the healing. I worked on Vanessa while conversing with Alejandro and May-Lee. Two days later, Juan called me from Vanessa's residence in Walnut Creek. His sister, he said, had left the hospital. Her temperature had suddenly dropped from 104 to 98.6. She felt so full of vitality that her intravenous hookups, no longer necessary, were disconnected, and she went home. He was elated.

I was satisfied. VQH is rapid, can successfully treat difficult cases, and is fully compatible with both Western and Eastern medicine. But I cautioned Juan that the physician's advice should still be followed. Vanessa continued with both conventional medical treatment and VQH, eventually leading to a complete remission of her cancer.

24. "Rediscovery is Every Bit as Good as Discovery"

While I cannot take credit for the discovery of the background material that follows, I have rediscovered a method of healing found in Jewish Scripture. Rediscovery is every bit as good as discovery when what is rediscovered is important and has been forgotten. It is better still when the rediscovered information has the capacity to improve the lives of those around us. According to the tradition of the Kabbalah, the *Torah* is written in a numerological code as well as in verse. Hebrew characters are all both numbers and letters. The following section explains how analysis of this numerological code leads to a healing process. *The Complete Book of Numerology* by Joyce Keller and Jack

Keller explains numerology in detail. With this inspiration from ancient wisdom and the modern science of VQH, I am convinced of the immense potential of applying this insight to the art of healing.

25. Background for the Four Phases

In VQH,

two Hebrew words are of great import:

***ruach* and *neshamah*.**

***Ruach* means air/energy/oxygen/spirit,**

and *neshamah* means breath/spirit/soul.

From Genesis 2:7, "And the Lord God formed man of the dust of the ground, and breathed into his nostrils the breath of life; and man became a living soul." The breath of life, *ruach*, and his soul, *neshamah*, came from God, from heaven. For the believer and nonbeliever alike, the rediscovery of the secret of life is within the scripture. However, faith in this belief system is not required to practice Visionary Quantum Healing.

I have further decoded these two Hebrew words. *Ruach* and *neshamah* are two of the three main words in the Bible (the third is *Nefesh*). They have roughly equivalent meanings, so insight into one word yields insight into the other two. Kabbalists are able to discern the deeper meanings of words by discovering sentences for which the word is an acronym. That is, the letters of the word under consideration appear as the initial letters of the words of a significant sentence that sheds light on the deeper meaning of the word. Thus, the single word serves as the code for the sentence, and the sentence serves to reveal the profound meaning of the word. The decoded letters of *Neshamah, Nun, Shin, Mem* and *Heh,* form the first letters of the sentence *"Nes sam mimarom Hashem"* ("Miracle established from Heaven by God").

The following is based on numerology. Information on numerological methods is available at http://en.wikipedia.org/wiki/numerology. Numerologists apply definitions to numbers. They use these definitions in conjunction with each other, to find the meaning of what ever they may be describing. Most numerological systems of today and in past human civilizations are formed from a base-10, or decimal system. Numerologists often reduce a number or word by a process known as digit summing. In the case of a number, you take the sum of all of the digits of the number, and if the result is a number with 2 or more digits you add up the digits of that number; you repeat the process recursively until you arrive at a single-digit number.

The Hebrew alphabet is a set of 22 letters used for writing the Hebrew language. Hebrew is written from right to left. The letters may also be used as numbers. This use of letters as numbers is used in Kabbalah (Jewish mysticism) in a practice known as Gemitraya. The Hebrew alphabet is thought to have developed in the same way as the Phoenician alphabet; each letter representing a picture. More information on the Hebrew alphabet is available at http://en.wikipedia.org/wiki/Hebrew_Alphabet.

As early as the 1st Century BCE Jews believed the Torah, first five books of the Bible, contained encoded message and hidden meanings. Gemitraya is one method for discovering hidden meanings in Torah. Each letter in Hebrew also represents a number. Hebrew, unlike many other languages, never developed a separate numerical alphabet. By converting letters to numbers, Kabbalists were able to find hidden meaning in each word. This method of interpretation was used extensively by various schools. An example would be the teachings of Rabbi Isaac Luria[1].

There is no one fixed way to "do" Gemitraya. Some say there are up to 70 different methods. One simple procedure is as follows: each syllable and/or letter forming a word has a characteristic numeric value. The sum of these numeric tags is the word's "key", and that word may be replaced in the text by any other word having the same key. Through the application of many such procedures, alternate or hidden meanings of scripture may be derived. Similar procedures are used by Islamic mystics, as described by Idries Shah in his book, *The Sufis.* More information on the Kabbalah and Gemitraya is available at http://en.wikipedia.org/wiki/Kabbalah

By applying a variety of Kabbalistic, numerological, geometric and algebraic analyses to the word *neshamah* and to the sentence *"Nes sam mimarom Hashem,"* I have discovered some fundamental insights into the nature of healing—specifically, why breath and air have such great healing power. Using the Kabbalistic practice of *Gematriya*, I computed that the numerical value of *nes* is 110, of *sam* is 340, of *mimarom* is 326, and of *Hashem* is 345. The sum total of these numbers is 1121, which is the numerical value of the entire sentence. Using another numerological system, I converted the number 1121 to a single-digit number by adding its digits. This conversion (1+1+2+1) yields the number 5, which signifies "communication" and is connected with the divine energy of *Gevurah* — "Strength." I also decided to perform numerological analyses on each word in the sentence. Thus, 110 (*nes*) becomes 2; 340 (sam) becomes 7; 326 (*mimarom*) becomes 11, which further reduces to 2; and finally 345 (*Hashem*) becomes 12, which further reduces to 3. Adding these numbers together, we get 14. Again, by adding the digits 1+4, this conversion yields the single digit number of 5. So either way we analyze these numbers, we arrive at 5, which again signifies "communication" and "*Gevurah* — Strength," the corresponding *Sefirot* in the Tree of Life shown in the diagram on page 83. If we add together the two 5s, we get 10, which signifies "abundance" and "*Malkhut* - Kingdom." Ten can be reduced to 1, which signifies "*Keter* - Crown" or "Divine Unity" (God). Furthermore, the *Gematriya* of the word *Neshamah* is 395. The 3 signifies "expansion" or "*Binah* - Understanding"; the 9 signifies "completion" or "*Yesod* - Foundation"; and the 5 signifies "communication" or "*Gevurah* - Strength." Moreover, the 395 can be converted to 17, which further reduces to 8. The "1" in "17" signifies "*Keter* - Crown" or "God," and the "7" signifies "*Netzach* - Internal Victory." Finally, 8 signifies "governance" as well as "*Hod* - Splendor" and magic.

נשמה , *neshamah* - breath, spirit or soul, 395 - 17 - 8 is

Governing Magic, 1 is G-d, 7 is internal victory.

English Word	Gemitraya	Kabbalah	Numerology
Miracle	110	נס	2
Establish	340	שם	7
From Heaven	326	ממרום	2, 11
By G-d	345	השם	3, 12
Total	1121		14
	5	Communication	5
5+5=10 Abundance			
10 Reduces to 1, symbolizing the Devine G-d			
Hands together, ask and you shall receive.			

Taken together, these complex analyses reveal that: 1) God is governing over the soul; 2) God gives the soul abundance and full strength to communicate with Him; and 3) the soul communicates with breath, air, happiness, wealth, health, magic, internal victory, expansion, and continuity.

I am grateful for the insights I have gained from the Kabbalah. As a late bloomer, I began taking Kabbalah courses in my early forties when I lived in New York City in the mid 1980s. The courses were offered at Stevenson High School. I can still remember a remarkable line from the *Zohar*, the Book of Splendor, that I learned at that time: When a man approaches his forties, he continues with his profession or goes back to complete his education. What perfect timing! I decided to commit myself to my education, and this commitment eventually led to my profession as a healer. After decades of investigating many different ways of healing, I concluded that most of the holistic and conventional approaches treated the symptoms, not the underlying causes. These approaches were expensive ways to achieve temporary relief, but did not offer real, long-lasting cures. The search for a real cure led me to the discovery of the process of Visionary Quantum Healing.

In the beginning, the seminal idea for VQH came from Scripture. As a boy of ten, I was at synagogue when a phrase from the morning service including the words *ruach* and *neshamah* spoke to me. The words felt so powerful that I was compelled to investigate further. After the prayer, I asked my father about the phrase that had caught my attention. Though he gave me an answer, something told me that there was more to it than he let on.

Perhaps my teacher would give me a different answer. I was right about that, but his answer did not seem complete, either. Possibly because I have been doing healing since I was five years old, this phrase spoke to me on a higher level. I guessed I was on to something, but I wasn't quite sure yet. I knew there must be someone who could give me the complete answer.

Weeks later, I mustered the chutzpah to ask the Rabbi about the meaning of *ruach* and *neshamah.* Rabbi Shalom had a very special way of expressing himself. Whenever he spoke, everyone listened attentively. No question was too big or too small for him. With kindness and patience, Rabbi Shalom took me aside. We sat on a bench while he conveyed the meaning of the phrase.

"You see, my son"— that's how he referred to his students, just as if we were part of his family — "*ruach* is "air/oxygen/energy/soul," *neshamah* is "breath, spirit or soul," so we are talking of a higher life. We know only of this life on earth according to Scripture. The *Torah* teaches us of the afterlife that is Eden. However, in The Book of Splendor (*Zohar*) we learn that there is a higher afterlife even above Eden; it is the life of the Righteous (*Tzaddik*). There are a few more afterlives that we don't know of—and then beyond that there is the highest one: God."

Since I loved the Rabbi and appreciated his wisdom, I thanked him for the lesson, and that lesson has stayed with me. However, from that day on, I have expanded upon the Rabbi's explanation, which I believe clarifies things. Although I have developed this theory through years of healing and research, the answer lies within the phrase itself.

After doing the extensive analyses described above, I concluded that air and soul are the "Miracle Established from Heaven by God." Air, oxygen, energy, soul and spirit are truly all one. It would be impossible to survive without them. If we just inhaled air, it would be impossible to live. If we just exhaled air, it would also be impossible to live. Since the air represents a great need of the soul, we can draw a crucial conclusion: Air/oxygen/energy/soul is the secret to life and the healing of the soul.

Later I experimented with the chakras. I combined and applied air and light energy to the front and back of the body, releasing it through the crown chakra. This led to an amazing transformation and a healing comfort to myself as well as clients. I found the healing on all levels to be rapid, satisfactory, and curative. With thirty-five years in the healing arts yielding great results and success, the testimonials of my clients speak clearly to both the immediate success and the long-term effects of this healing process.

Thus, I have established an experiential basis for this remarkable healing work. By applying a reciprocating motion with the palm of the hand, with the hand facing down, parallel, and in close proximity to the skin of a client, a soothing, healing effect is produced in the area. A reciprocating hand motion of approximately two to five cycles per second produces a small movement of air between the hand and the client's body; an upward movement creates a slight vacuum that draws the air under the hand and then up and away. In this way the healer can slowly move his or her hand over portions of the body with an up-and-down motion perpendicular to the body until the client feels total relief in the area of discomfort. The whole process usually takes about 15 to 20 minutes. I will describe and illustrate these approaches in Chapter Four, the Four Phases of Visionary Quantum Healing.

As a scientist, a healer, and a man of faith, I am confident that this phrase including the words *ruach* and *neshamah* from the Hebrew Scripture holds the secret to healing as well as to the life of the soul. I'm also led to believe that I have developed a method that works under any conditions, one that is truly different and really effective, and that any student, client or practitioner can learn to do it by following the Four Phases. A common question is if VQH works both during the day and night. As discussed in "Genesis and Light," page 41, there are two great lights, the greater for the day and the lesser for night, providing natural light for healing at any time.

My hope is that in the near future, this method will eventually replace not only all other existing holistic methods, but most conventional ones as well — for they are expensive, unreliable, and often ineffective. In contrast, VQH leads the way to the future. The students who have practiced the Four-Phase Healing Process tell of great success.

The Four Phases of Visionary Quantum Healing™

Chapter Four

The Process

26. Phase I: Relaxation and Feeling the Depth of Pain

To my knowledge, there are no clients who would not benefit from the treatment presented here. I specialize in difficult problems, physical as well as emotional.

The session is divided into three or four treatments, that last two to three minutes each, until the client reports a pain level of zero. There is no set timetable. Everything depends on how long it takes to dissipate the foreign entities and how much healing energy the client's body draws in with each treatment. Once the client's body

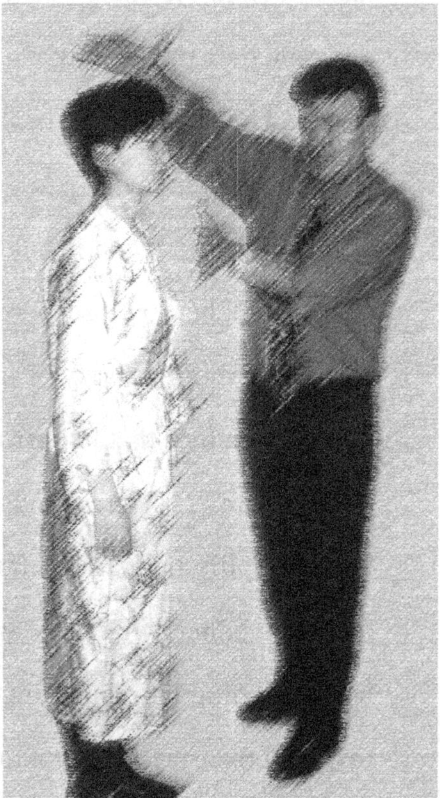

Phase I

This artist's conception shows the pervasive unseen energy flowing all around healer and client. Allow the legs to be the sole support for the body.

has drawn in the energy it needs, I move my hands more quickly and conclude the healing.

This first set of five illustrations applies to the first five steps of the treatment.

The client and I stand facing each other, about five feet apart. I ask her to close her eyes and allow her legs to be the sole support of her body. I then ask her to feel her suffering and rate the depth of that pain from zero to ten — ten being the most intense pain. If she responds with a number less than ten, I tell her to amplify the pain as much as possible so that she can easily feel and connect with it. With my hands, I bounce a laser-like beam of natural air and light energy over the chakras, bouncing my hand over the first chakra and slowly moving on to the next, with a reciprocal motion in a direction perpendicular to the palm. By amplifying her pain, the client can feel the changes and relief more immediately and dramatically. This heightened awareness of pain creates an incentive for the client to continue the healing process into the next phase.

Phase 1 Step 1

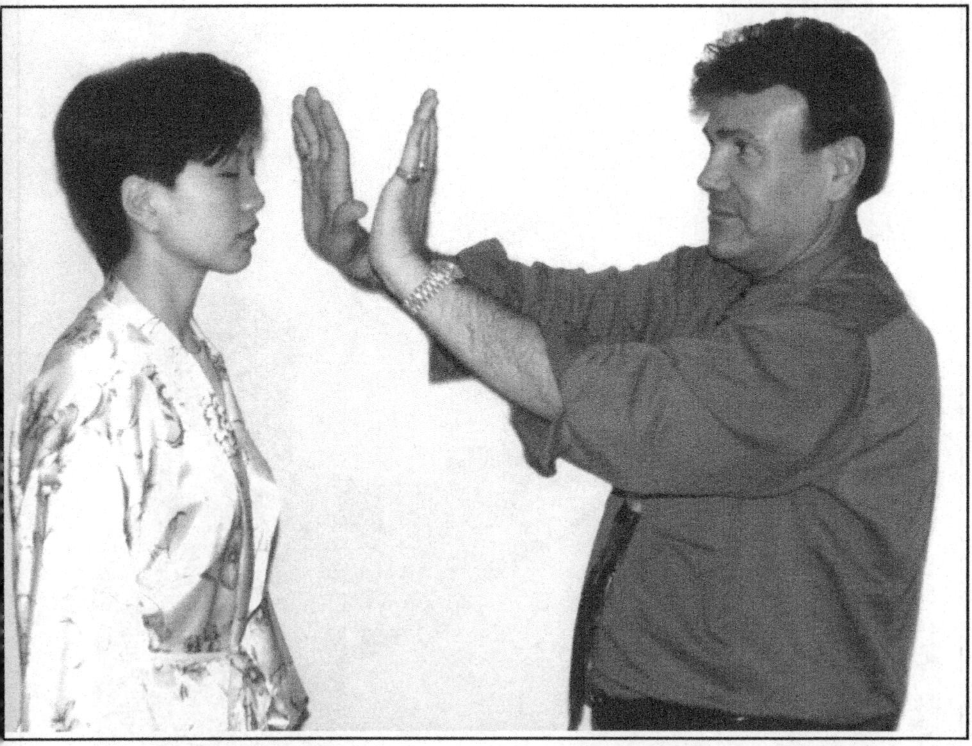

While the client's eyes remain closed, the Visionary Healer begins transmitting a laser-like beam back and forth.

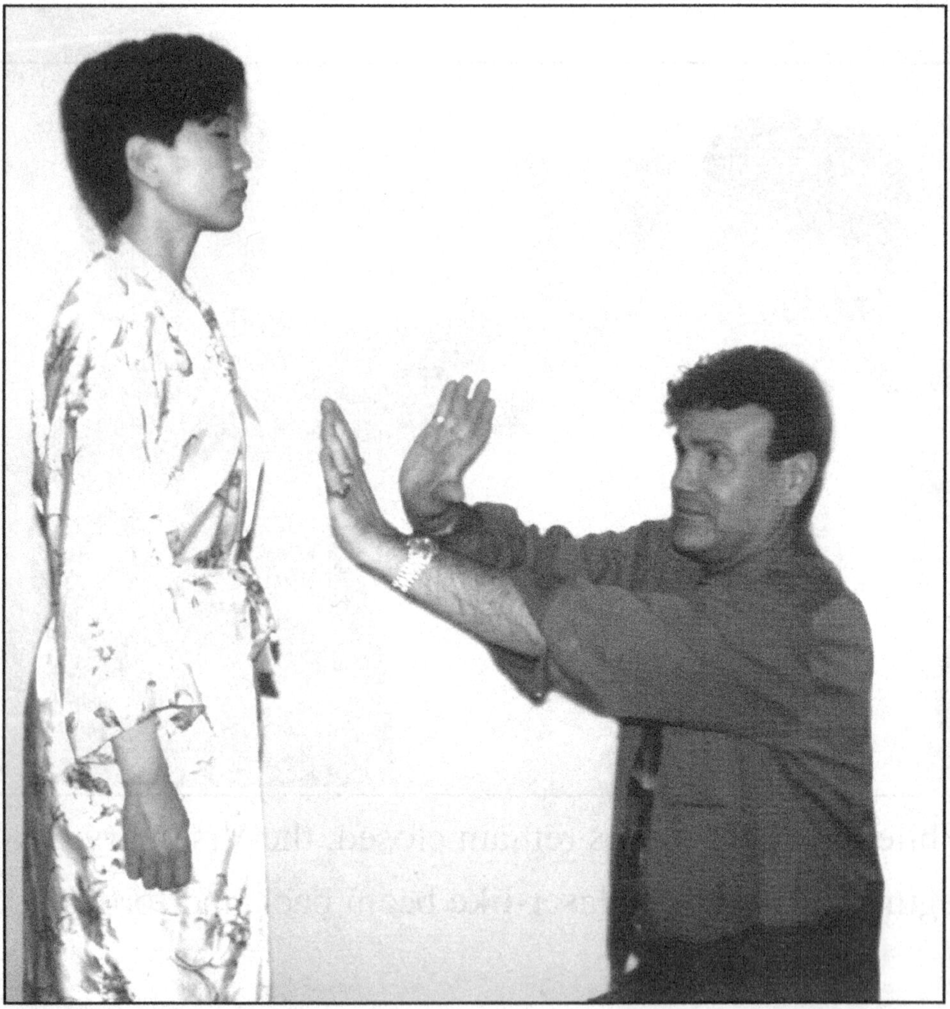

Using a back and forth motion, the Visionary Healer inundates the client with the full force of natural air and light energy.

Phase 1 Step 3

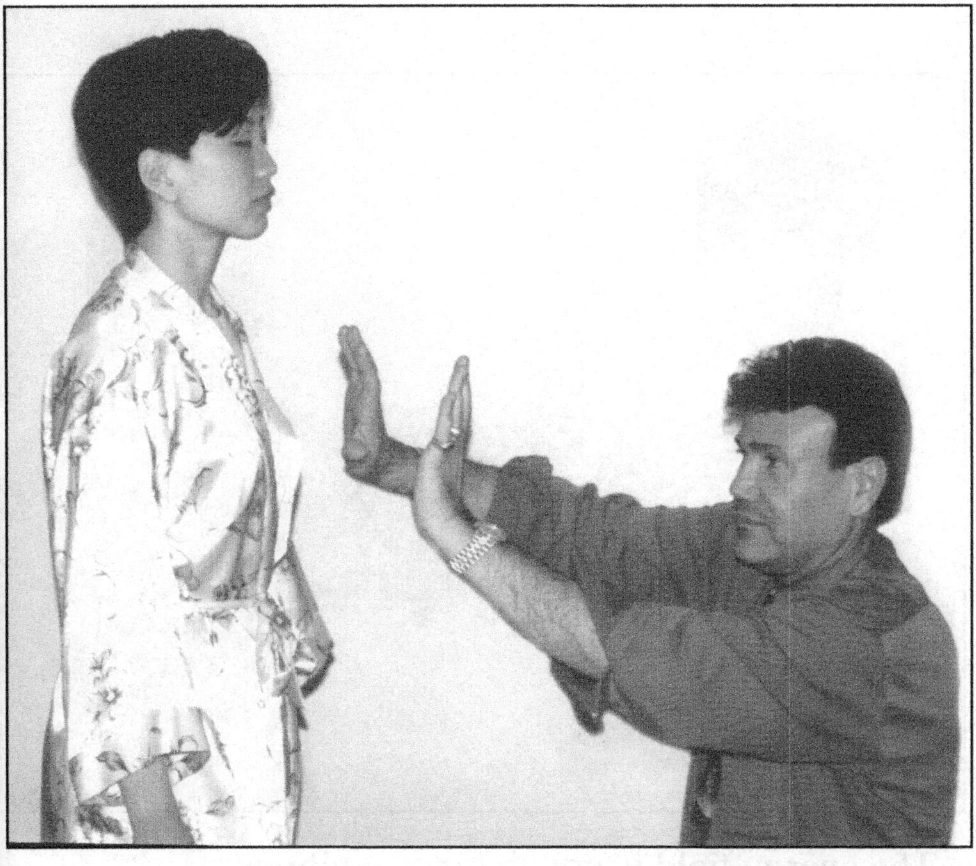

The Visionary Healer uses the energy that gathers from the surrounding natural air and light energy field.

Phase 1 Step 4

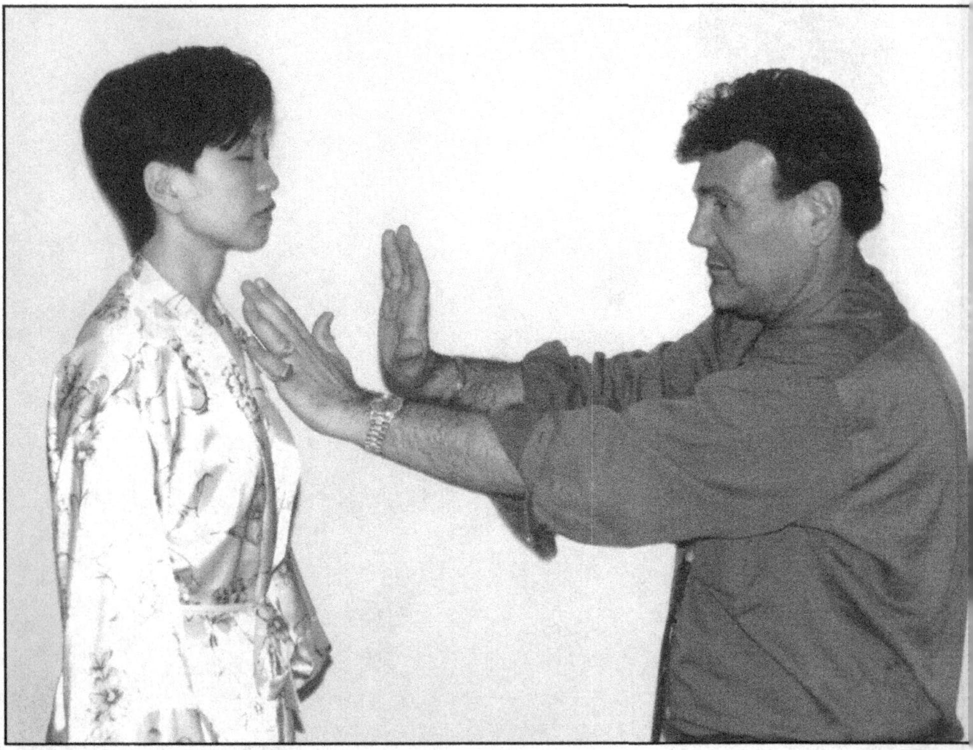

The energy field is now intensely vibrant.

Phase 1 Step 5

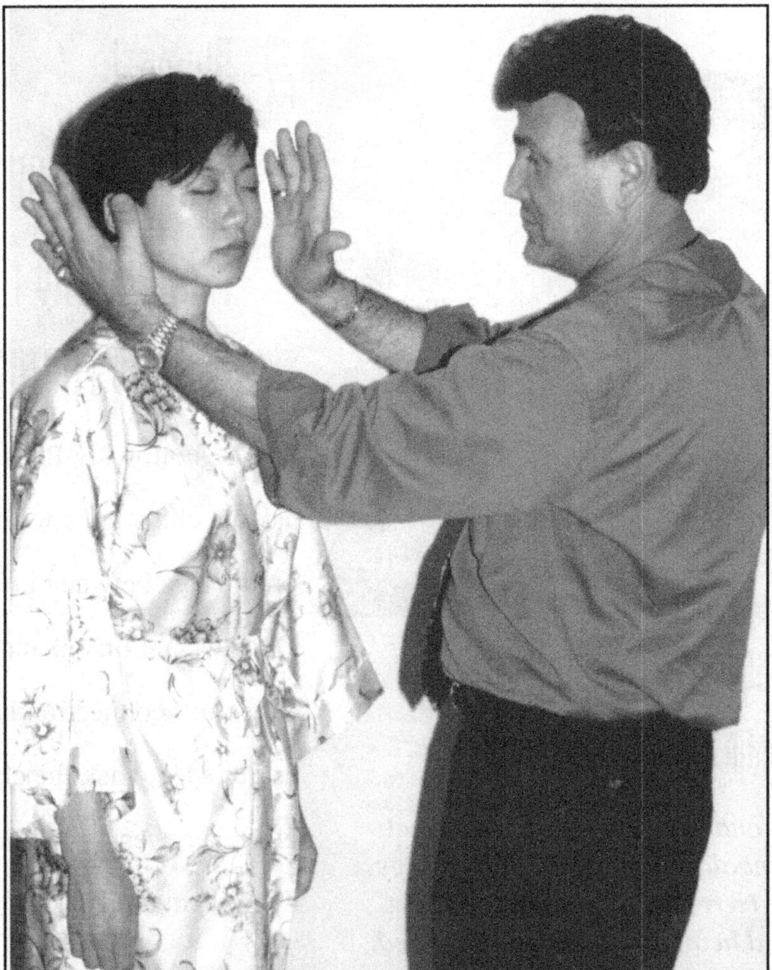

Gradually moving higher, the Visionary Healer bounces the natural air, light and healing energy back and forth over the client's face and ears.

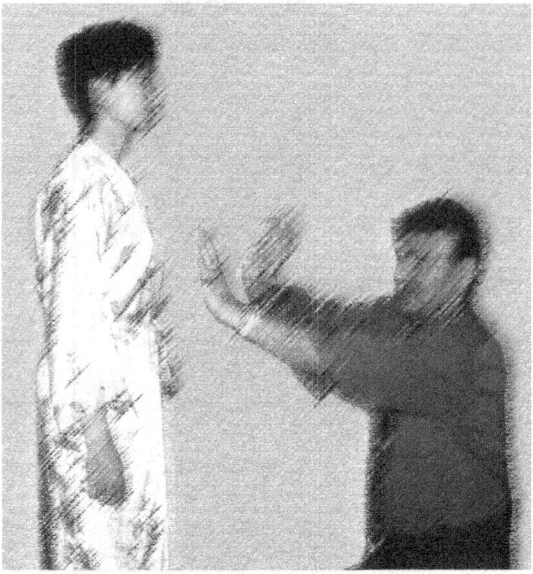

With my hands, I bounce a laser-like beam back and forth.

A Visionary Healer learns to detect any imbalance in the client's energy field. Here, the unseen energy flow around healer and client is depicted.

27. Phase 2: Concentration and Establishing the Healing Energy Link

Following Phase 1, I ask the client to concentrate on the area between my eyes. Once we are linked and the conscious connection is clearly established, I ask the client to close her eyes again and not open them until asked. VQH research indicates that healing is most effective if the client's eyes remain closed during the process.

In Phase 2, I put one hand, palm down, over the crown chakra, and with my other hand continually bounce laser-like beams of natural air, light, and healing energy, gradually moving higher, cleansing one chakra at a time. The healing will not be complete until the client reaches a pain level of zero.

Phase 2 Step 1

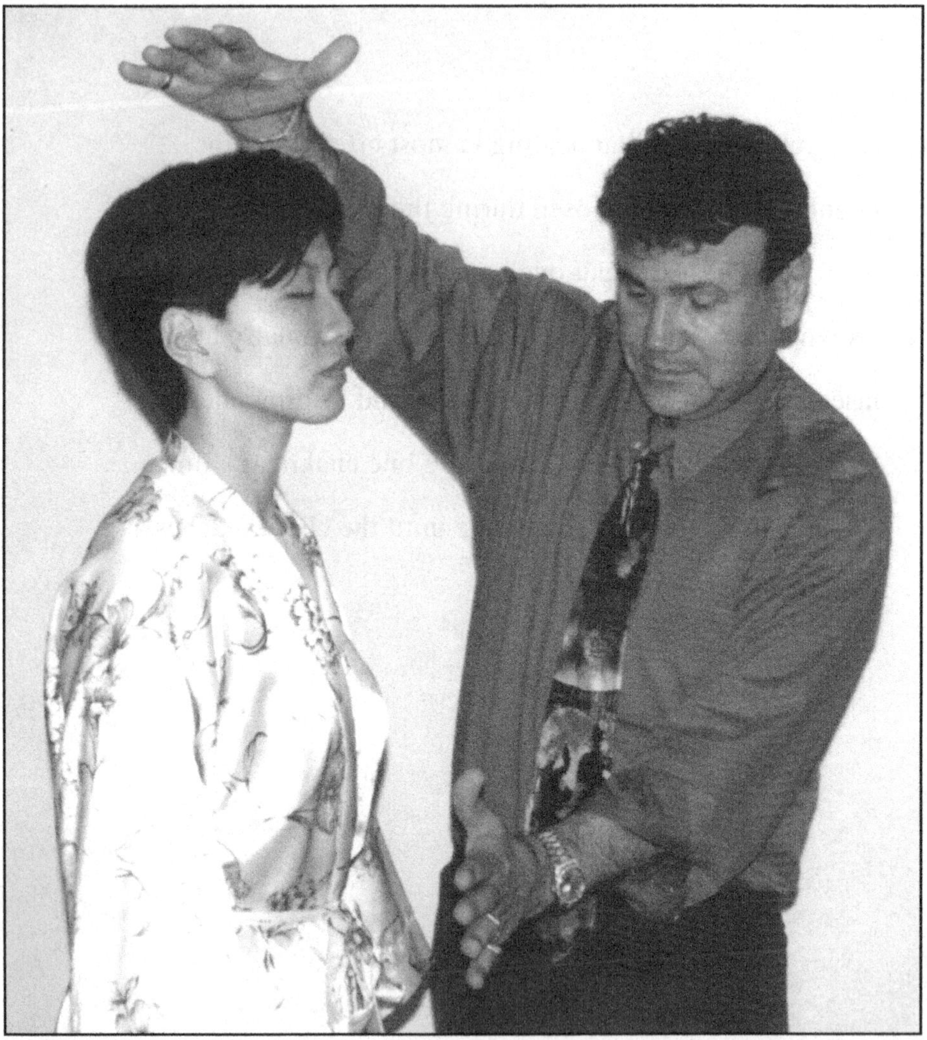

The Visionary Healer delivers three reciprocal motions with the full force of both hands while moving the natural air, light, and healing energy back and forth.

Phase 2 Step 2

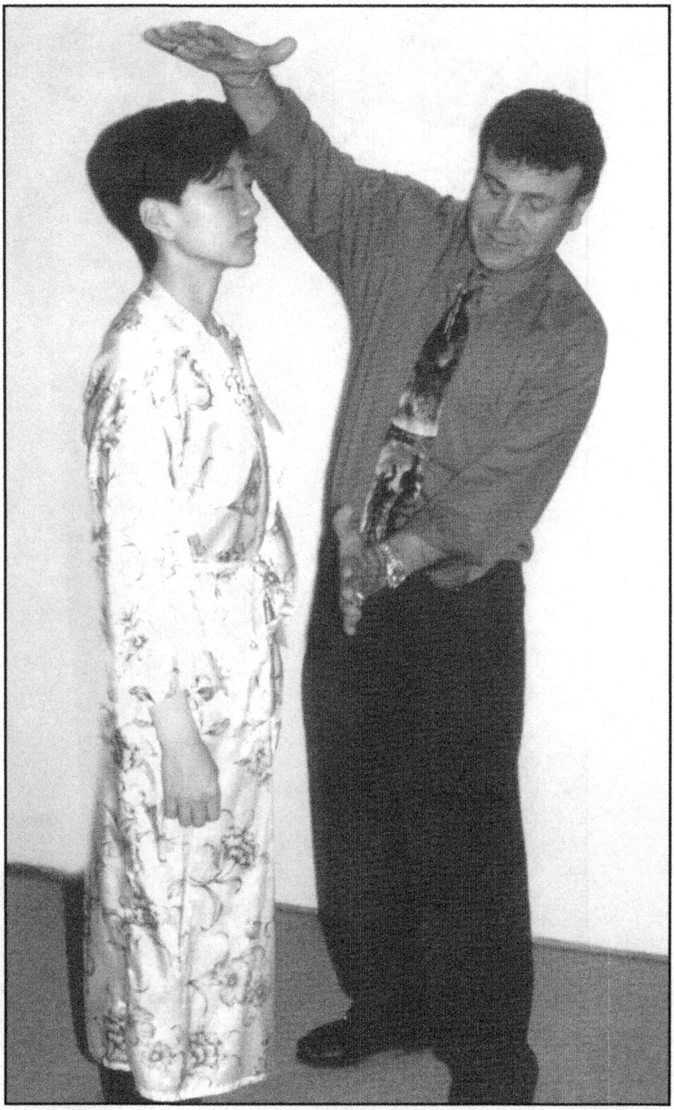

The Visionary Healer cleanses one chakra at a time, gradually moving from lower to higher.

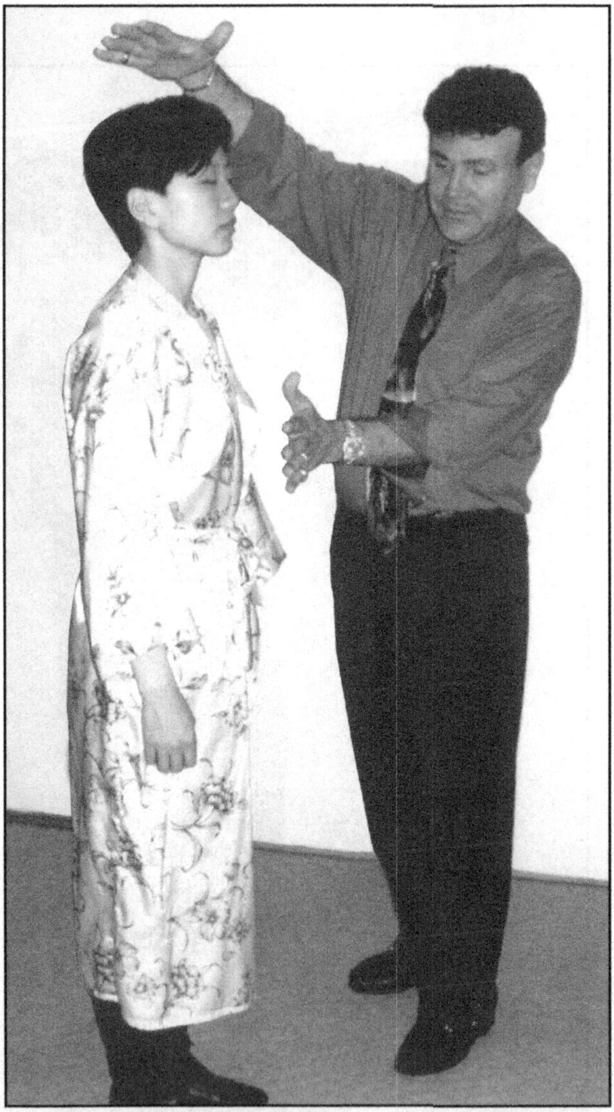

The Visionary Healer gradually moves his left hand from lower to higher chakras while the right hand remains hovering over the crown chakra.

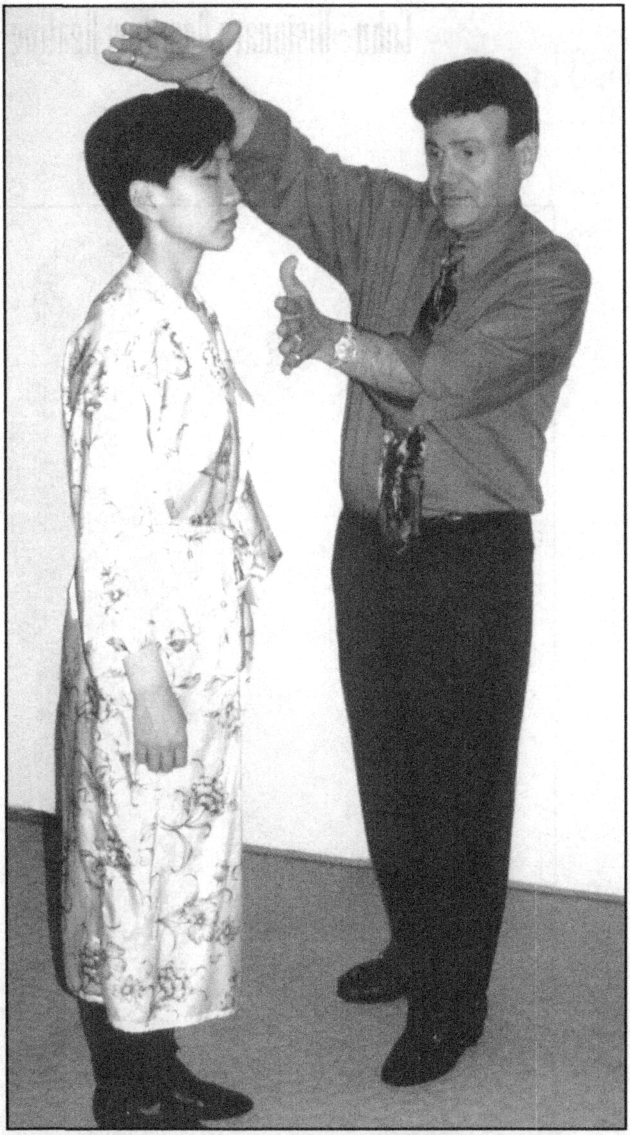

The Visionary Healer continuously bounces a laser-like beam of natural air, light, and healing energy back and forth toward the crown chakra.

Phase 2 Step 5

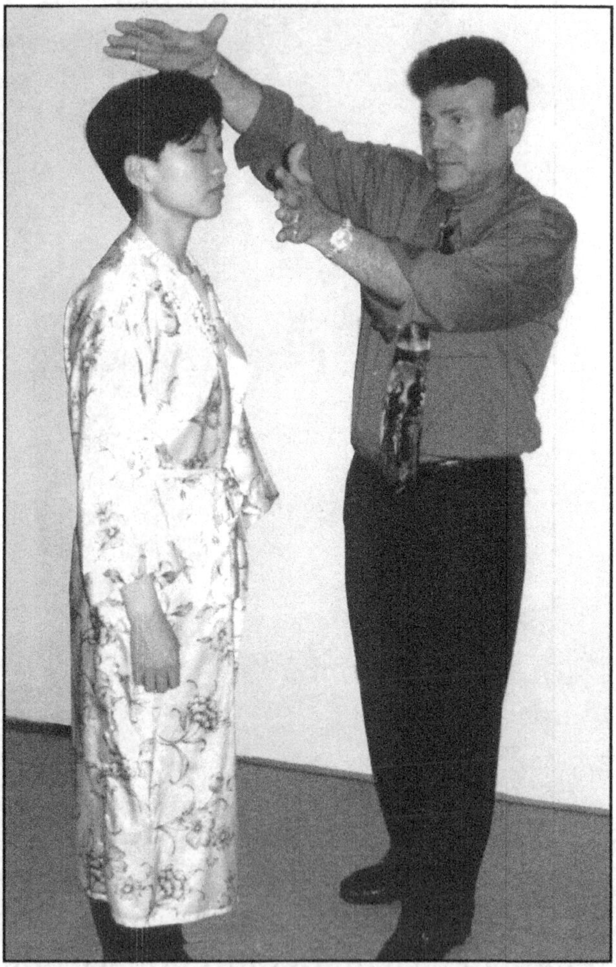

The cleansing motion is repeated through all the chakras, on the front of the body.

28. Phase 3: Healing with Pure Natural Air, Light, and Healing Energy

While the client's eyes remain closed, I continue transmitting a laser-like beam of natural air, light, and healing energy, back and forth, perpendicular to her body, inundating her with the full force of the energy. This energy field, often called the aura, is now intensely vibrant. It is significant that the word "aura" literally means "air, breeze, wind." This phase takes three to five minutes.

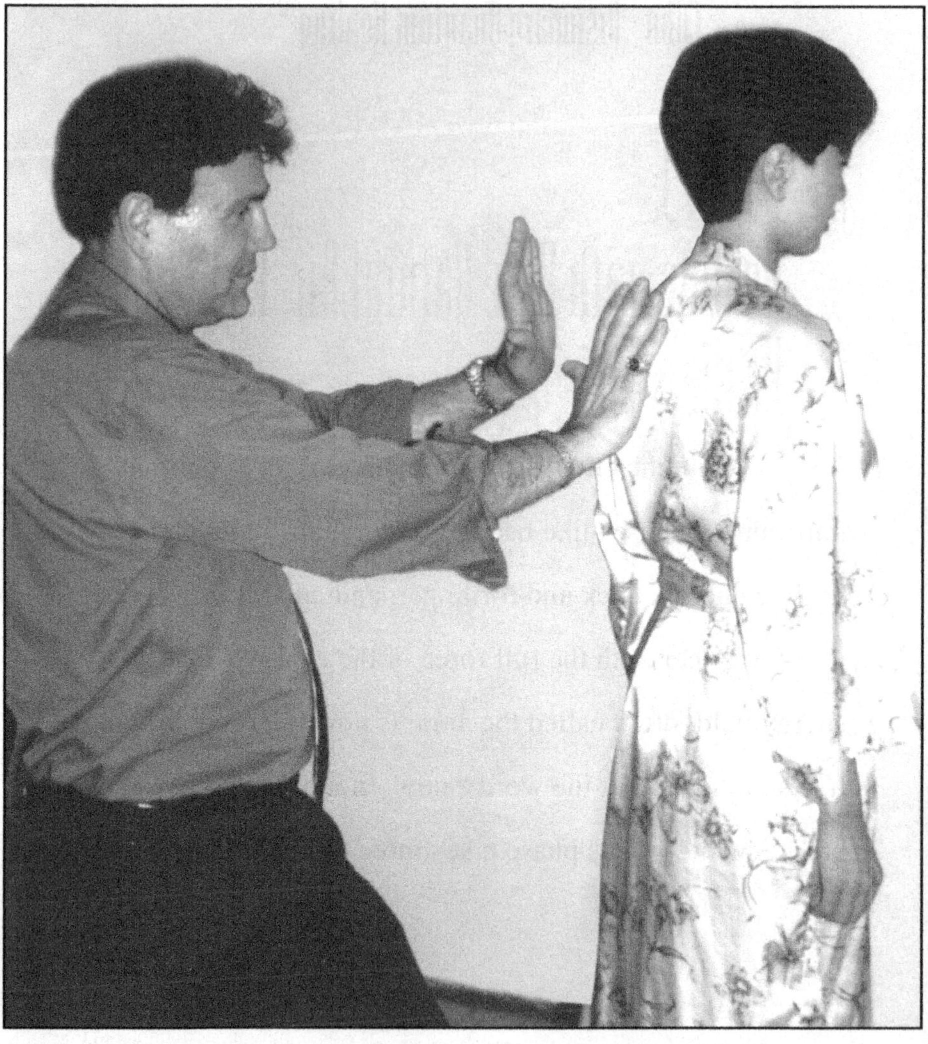

With the full force of natural air, light, and healing energy, the Visionary Healer bounces a laser-like beam back and forth through the chakras, perpendicular to the back of the body.

Phase 3 Step 2

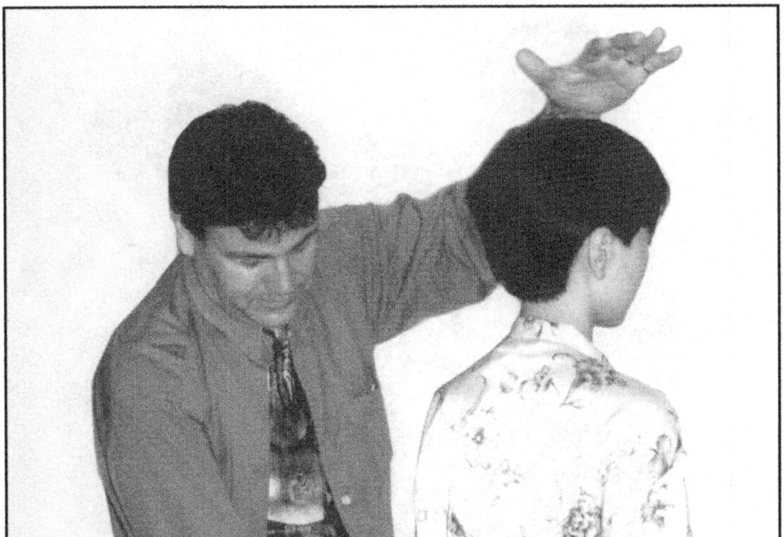

The Visionary Healer again begins with the lowest chakra, right hand with palm down, left hand hovering over the crown chakra.

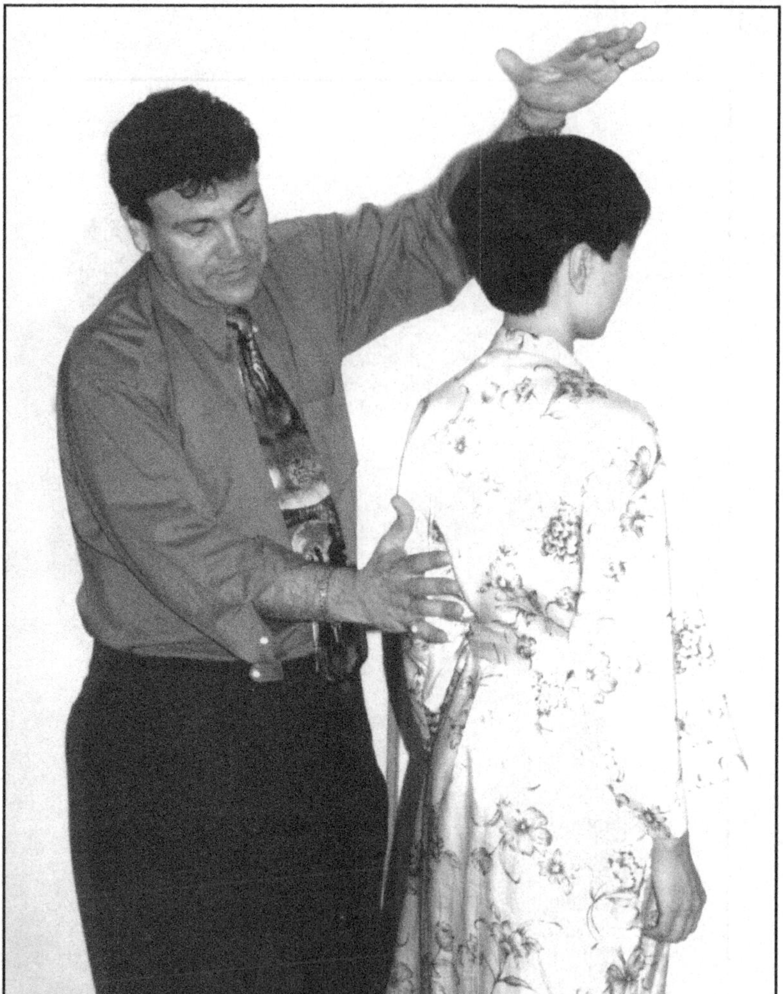

The Visionary Healer's right hand gradually moves higher, cleansing one chakra at a time with three repetitions.

Phase 3 Step 4 Cohn - Visionary Quantum Healing™

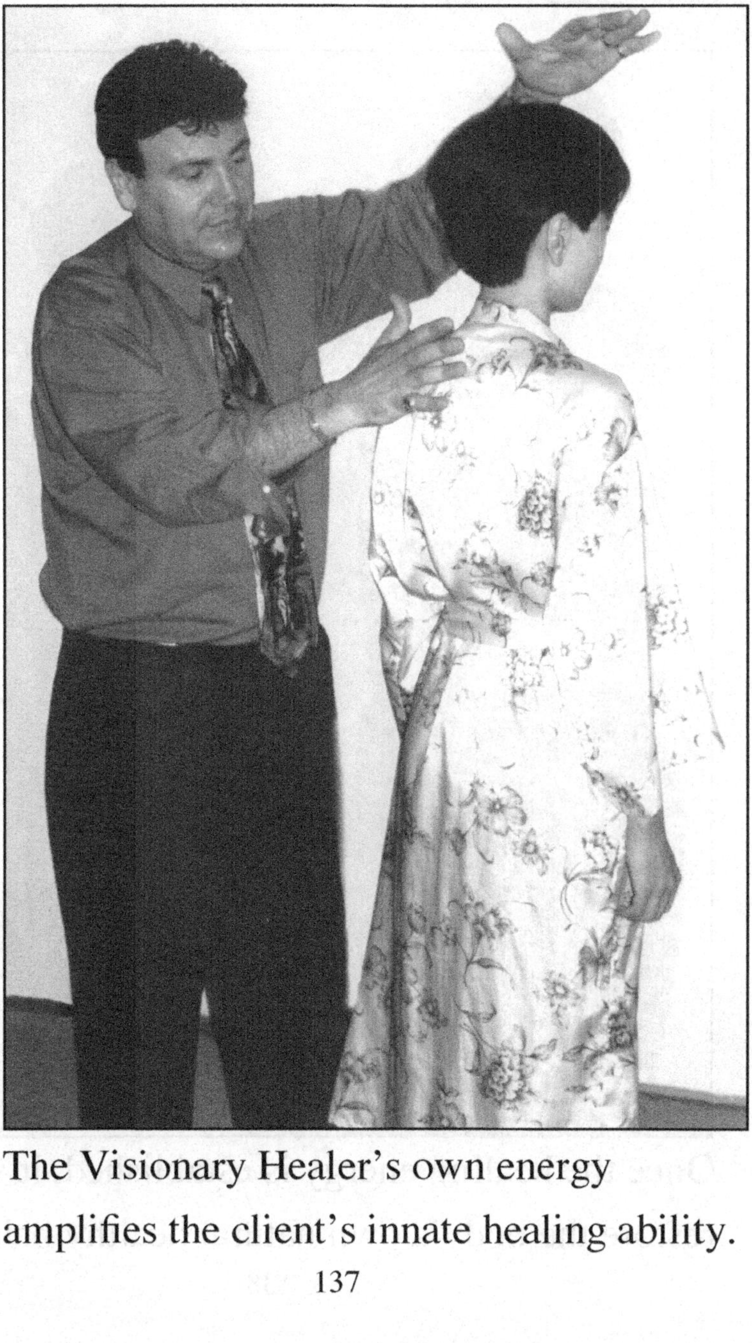

The Visionary Healer's own energy amplifies the client's innate healing ability.

Phase 3 Step 5

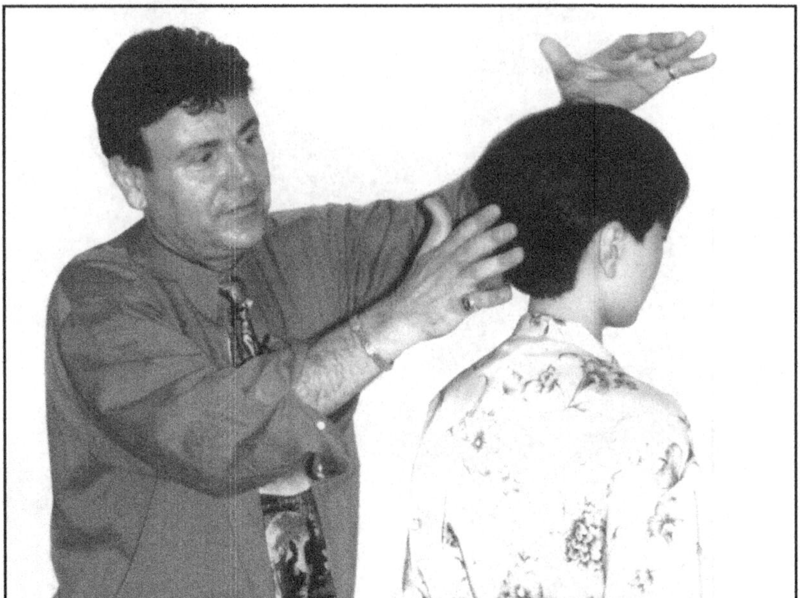

Once the healing energy is established, it will restore the body's own natural healthy balance.

29. Phase 4: Cleansing the Body and the Seven Chakras

Within this phase, there are five steps. First, using both of my hands, I bounce a laser-like beam of natural air, light, and healing energy back and forth, perpendicular to the body, initially over the client's chest, then over the seven chakras, beginning with the lowest.

When this is completed, I start the second step: I place one hand, palm down, hovering over the crown chakra, while the other hand is bouncing the laser-like beams beginning with the lowest chakra.

Third, I gradually move higher, cleansing one chakra at a time, doing three repetitions on each chakra.

Fourth, from the lowest chakra and using the full force of both hands, I direct the beam upward and bounce it back and forth over the client's face and ears. Moving from the lower torso upward, the hands generate beams that engulf the shoulders and spine. In this last step, I purge the internal and external foreign entities, the diseases.

The Fourth Phase is the final dispersal of the foreign entities and self-cleansing. The diseases disperse completely, vanishing out of the crown chakra. I move away and speak: "Open your eyes. What pain level do you feel now?"

Normally, if the client started at level ten, she may reply that she is at six or seven. I reassure the client that she is making progress. How quickly the client will reach zero varies. It is very important for the healer to understand that the client is only healed when the rating approaches zero, which indicates total elimination of the entities and pain. The healer may have to repeat the process after a couple of minutes, and will need to exercise patience.Before the client leaves, I let him or her relax, drink liquids and rest.

Phase 4 Step 1

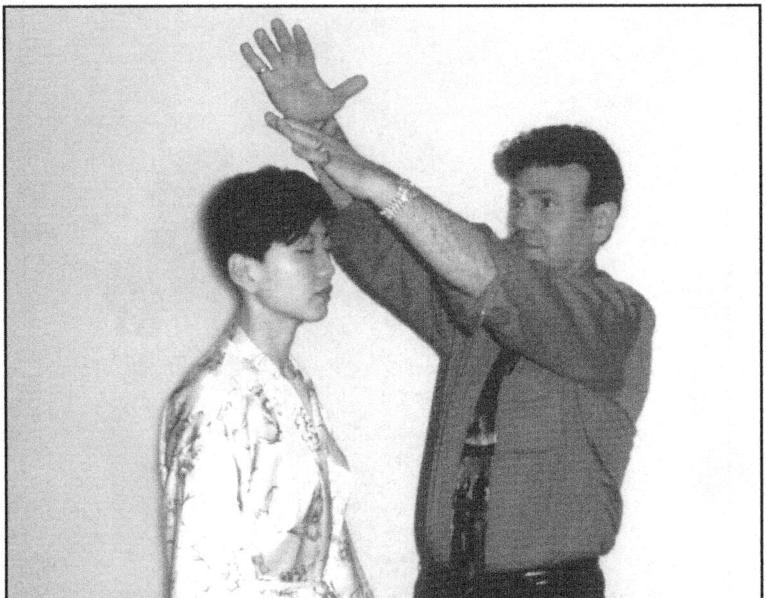

With the full force of both hands, the Visionary Healer bounces the foreign entities out of the crown chakra.

Phase 4 Step 2

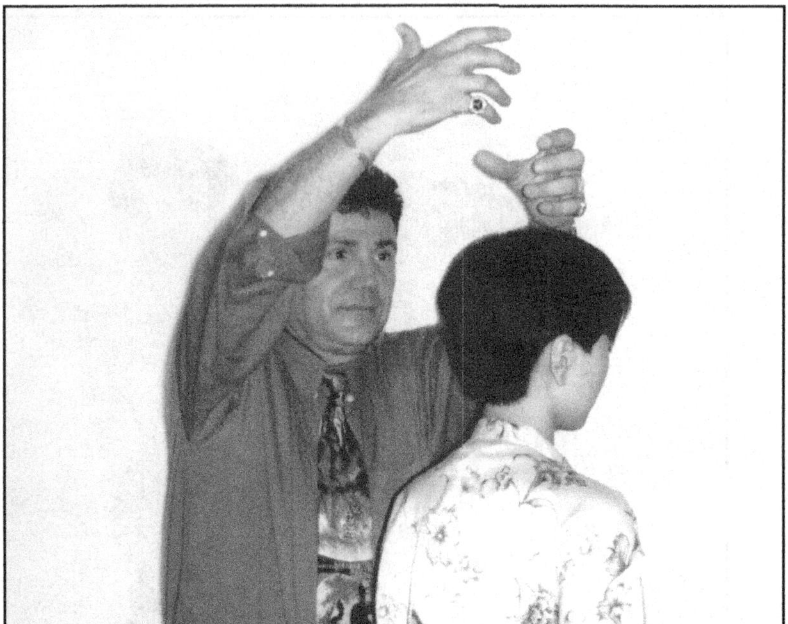

The Visionary Healer evaporates the foreign entities out of the crown chakra.

Phase 4 Step 3

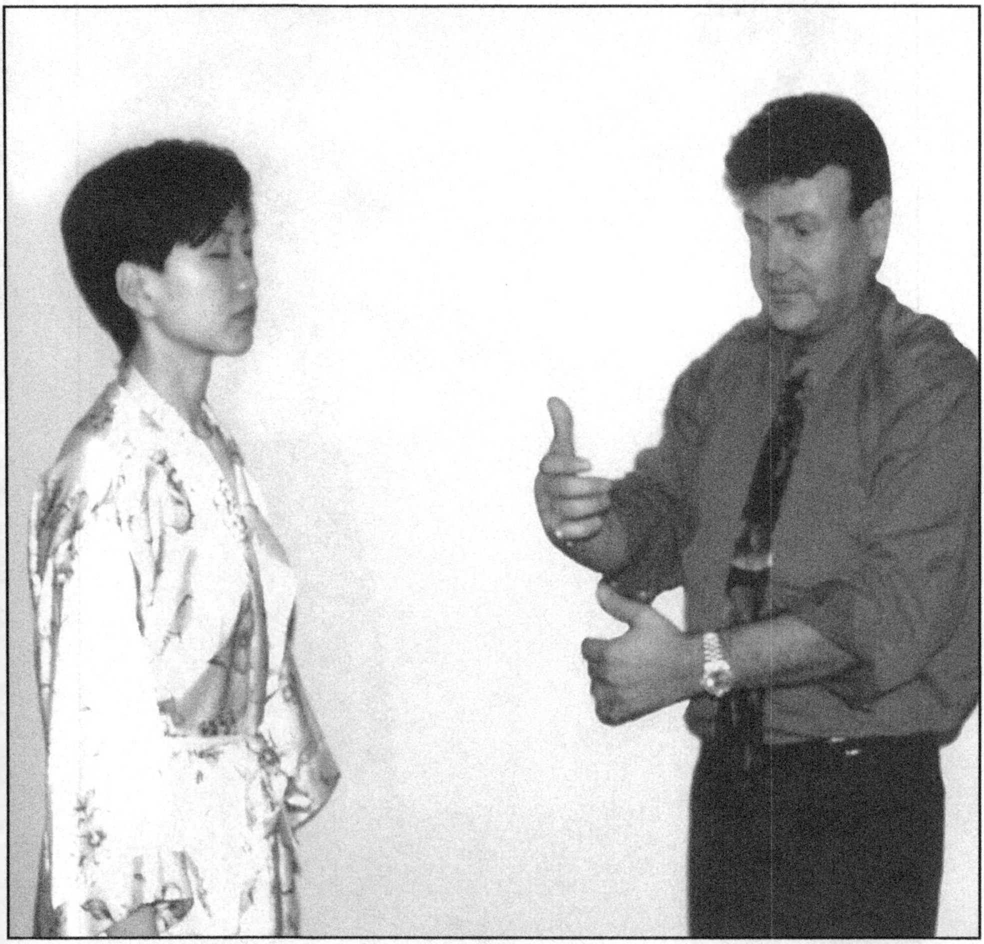

After each treatment, the Visionary Healer always protects himself to regain his energy.

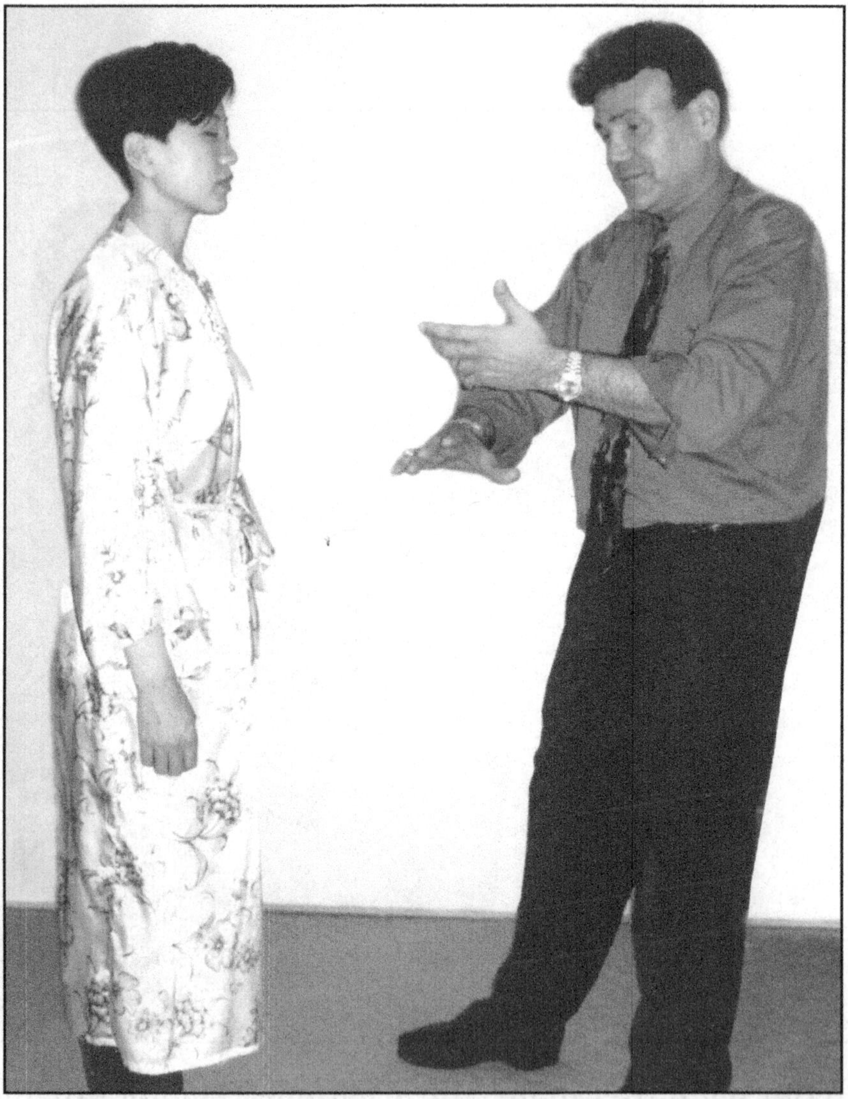

The Visionary Healer immediately protects himself by cutting an imaginary rope around his neck and his waist with his hand.

30. Aftermath: Protection and Restoring Potency

It is important to remember that many clients have exhausted all forms of conventional and holistic treatments and so may have very strong foreign entities in them. After administering treatment, I immediately protect myself. When the disease is released into the astral realm, it may try to invade the healer. As soon as I finish with the client, I make sure to replenish my energy. The protective process I use involves imaging a rope around my neck and around my waist that is connected to the client. I then use my right (dominant) hand to cut the rope and completely sever my energetic connection with the client, repeating the process one to four times. From many other respected healers, I have learned that the healer can, if not careful, pick up harmful energy from clients.

31. The Qualified Practitioner: Mere Imitation Could Be Deadly

In India, people tell the story of a farmer whose horse was suffering from a huge bulge in its throat. The veterinarian was called, and after examining the horse's neck, he asked for a mallet. He whacked the horse in the neck and the bulge disappeared. Everyone was amazed.

However, a few weeks later, a huge bulge appeared on the other side of the horse's neck. This time the farmer thought, "Why pay the doctor? I saw what he did last time." So he took a mallet and whacked the horse, which collapsed and died.

The doctor was called to explain the horse's mysterious death. Incensed, the veterinarian explained,

"When I was here last, I examined the horse and noticed he had a squash stuck in his throat. So I crushed it with the mallet, and he was able to swallow again. But this time, your horse was suffering from goiter. The blow from your mallet killed him!"

From this story we learn the necessity of carefully training others to qualify them as Visionary Quantum healers. As a Visionary Quantum Healing practitioner with decades of experience and a strong academic background, I am committed to educating, training, and qualifying students to heal others as well as themselves. When healing is done improperly, it can backfire on the healer. Healers must be properly trained or read this book to learn how to restore their energy immediately. Imitation can be deadly, and it is also deadly to operate on false premises.

This underscores the importance to clients, students, and practitioners interested in doing VQH of reading this book and/or attending my seminar to learn how to safely practice this method of healing. A certificate as a Qualified Practitioner of Visionary Quantum Healing is available to those who complete the seminar or finish reading this book.

Chapter Five *The History*

32. A Child's Gift

Not only was my Mother an Orthodox Jew, but she was also the granddaughter of the Righteous Rabbi Chaiim Pinto. People from all over the world visited my mother to receive her healing prayers. Mother was able to heal other people, but when it came to healing herself, she would pray and seek the blessing of her late grandfather. For example, she suffered from unbearable migraines, but her prayers for relief seemed to go unanswered. Then one night, when I was five years old, she had a dream in which Rabbi Chaiim Pinto revealed to her, "You have heaven's gift right in your home."

She was bewildered and cried, "Where?"

"Salomon. Take his hand, place it on your forehead, and you will be healed."

This worked for Mother, and so she used to bribe me with candies and bring suffering neighbors to the house to have me heal them. Since it would be many years before I developed Visionary Quantum Healing, I used a hands-on method. I have been distributing "heaven's gift" to believers and nonbelievers alike since that time.

I am often asked if I was born a healer or if I was transformed into one by traumatic experience, chronic illness, or a life-threatening event. Though heredity and trauma have both played a part, I believe that we all, to different degrees, are born with healing abilities. For a while, although my family background pointed me in that direction, even I was unaware of my own ability as a healer.

My Mother spent her life healing others, even those well beyond our family, with her power of prayer. Ours was a family with a great lineage of healers. It was my Mother who, from the beginning, always told me that I had been given a special gift. She told me never to fear anything that might occur in my mind while healing anyone, for I would be protected, both as a healer and as a person.

She also taught me how to regain my healing energy after healing someone, by drinking a glass of water after each session. In addition, she cautioned me to be careful and to do the healing properly and sincerely. I now know these things from my practical experience in healing, but when I reflect on how my Mother revealed my healing abilities, I am eternally grateful to her. She put me on the right path.

If it were not for my Mother, I might have never fully realized that I possess this gift, and my life might have turned out quite differently. Today, I understand my ability to see, feel, and understand things that are not what we normally consider part of the "healing world." All human beings have the right to be healed.

33. Healing and the Six-Day War

In 1967, during the Six-Day War, when Syria, Lebanon, Jordan, and Egypt attacked Israel, my battalion had to fight the Egyptian commandos. When our armored vehicle was ambushed at Jabbel Libney in the middle of the Sinai Desert, I was twice hit by shrapnel, and a fellow soldier was shot in the throat. With blood flowing profusely over both of us, I held my hands on his neck to stop the blood flow for half an hour until the paramedics arrived. Only then did I attend to the wounds in my leg. For both his wounds and mine, I used my hands, for at this time I was still a hands-on healer. But I did have an uncanny healing touch: my leg sealed itself within a week or so, without surgery.

My companion's recovery was equally miraculous. After the war, I was invited to the kibbutz wedding of an officer, who was a friend. There I met the fallen soldier again, and he was fine — completely healed. He thanked me for helping to save his life. I told him, "Don't thank me. Your name saved you." His name was *Ezra*, which means "help" in Hebrew. Names *can* be prophetic of our calling in life.

34. Learning from My Own Dreams

In 1994, I was strolling with a colleague in

downtown San Francisco. A young Hasidic Jew approached us with cassette tapes, books, and a *Jewish Encyclopedia.* The cassette was about the interpretation of dreams according to *Kabbalah.* As usual, I gave a donation and accepted the tape. We shook hands as I thanked him.

The information on the tape really caught my interest and I listened to it incessantly — both in my car and at home. It prompted me to study primary source materials on dream interpretation and symbolism. When I dreamed, I recorded and interpreted my own dreams. More importantly, I gained insight into my gift to heal. This "chance" meeting with the young Orthodox Jew (*Chabadnic*) deepened my connection to my personal and ancestral pasts and encouraged my commitment to the healing world.

Gradually I became adept in dream interpretation.

Once, on the eve of *Shavuot*, I had an extraordinary dream that forever changed my life. *Shavuot* is the Jewish holiday that celebrates the giving of the *Torah* to the Jewish people on Mount Sinai. As a result of my dream, I now believe in the predetermined course of events. The *Talmud* considers *Shavuot* a concluding holiday to Passover and even refers to it by the name *Atzeret*, meaning "conclusion." Also known as the beginning "Feast of the Harvest" and "Festival of the First Fruits," it marks the preparatory time before Moses received the Ten Commandments on Mount Sinai. Each of the Jewish festivals holds special significance as an event to be observed as specified by God in the Torah.

At this point I had stopped doing healing for some time, because I was unsure of my rate of success and was concerned about the long-term efficacy of the healing. In

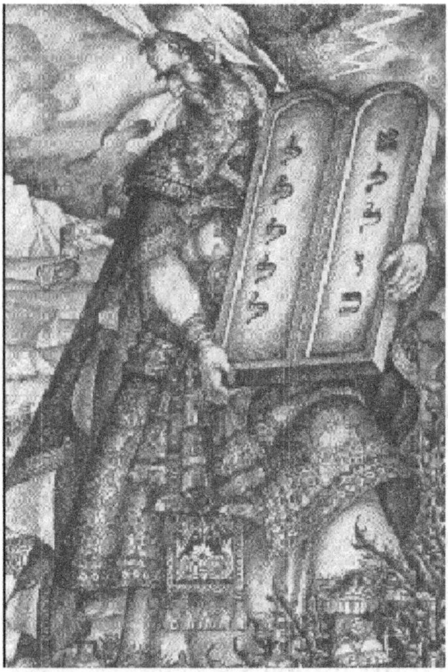

Moses receives the Ten Commandments. 3,313 years later he commands me to "Heal the suffering."

my dream I was walking in a marketplace in Egypt with Moses. This dream occurred in 1994, around May 5th or 6th, which is Sivan 5754, according to the Hebrew calendar. Moses was a very tall and imposing figure, dressed in white garb with golden trim and with golden sandals strapped to his feet. He put his arm around me and said, "Salomon, why don't you place your hand upon people and heal them from their suffering?" I looked up, smiling. "Moses, I have been doing this my whole life. You're not telling me anything new."

"Salomon, just lay your hands upon people, pray for them," he implored, "and they will be healed. And you will be truly gratified and fulfilled." I awoke ecstatic and in tears. Unsure if I was dreaming or having a vision, I said to myself, "What an *incredible* dream!"

This was a command that has not been hard to keep. The dream caused me to focus on concluding my education and continuing my quest for the development of the healing art that is now called Visionary Quantum Healing.

35. From the Tehilim (Psalms) of King David

That afternoon, in downtown San Francisco, I chanced upon Rami, a friend who had renewed his faith in religion. For some reason I felt comfortable revealing my dream to him. He was genuinely impressed and invited me to the synagogue for the Shavuot celebration that evening. I told him that attending shul for the high holidays - Rosh Hashana and Yom Kippur - was enough for me. But he convinced me and I agreed to go. I arrived at the synagogue around 8:30 that evening. The synagogue was packed with people in joyous celebration.

From across the room, I saw a hand waving, motioning me to come over. It was difficult to make my way through the crowd. I sat down next to Rami; on my other side was the Rabbi. I said to Rami, "Did you pay for this seat?" He said, "God sat you here. While everyone is singing and feasting, tell the Rabbi your dream."

I told Rabbi Ezran of my dream. He was very pleased and said, "Act on it!" Around midnight, when the congregation began leaving the synagogue, the Rabbi implored them to stay and continue celebrating such an auspicious occasion. Shavuot is of special significance to Sephardic Jews. According to our tradition, one should sit in the synagogue and read the Psalms of King David, the *Book of Tikkun-Olam* (The Healing of the World), and the *Book of Talmud* (the authoritative body of Jewish tradition). The Psalms say that both King David and his son, King Salomon, were born and died on *Shavuot.*

Of course most people, even the Rabbi, had family commitments. However, a mysterious compulsion made me volunteer to stay. So I approached the Rabbi and asked if I could stay the night reading the *Tehilim* (Psalms). He looked puzzled.

"You will stay here all night by yourself ?"

"Rabbi, is this not the house of God? Then should I be afraid?"

"No. No! Of course not."

"All right — then I'll stay, reading throughout the night."

Alone in the shul, I opened a Hebrew book and read *Tikkun Olam*, paying special attention to some verses I had been taught by my late father. Then I opened the Psalms of King David and began to read aloud, well into the early morning hours. I read the entire book, except for the first page, which was in print too small to read, kissed it, and walked up to the Ark where the *Torah* scroll is kept. I kissed the Ark door as well, and prayed for my children and family, and for world health, security, wisdom, and peace.

I opened the Psalms once again to the first page, yet still couldn't read it, even with my reading glasses. Then, magically, a gigantic page appeared before my eyes. I read it, then kissed the *Torah* and the Psalms and moved away from the Ark. As a former magician acquainted with all sorts of illusions, I was bewildered as I unsuccessfully tried to find the source of the giant page.

As I was about to leave, people began entering the synagogue for morning prayers.

"Salomon, where are you going?"

"Home."

"Stay with us for *Minyon Shavuot Shacharit* (early morning prayer). It will do you good."

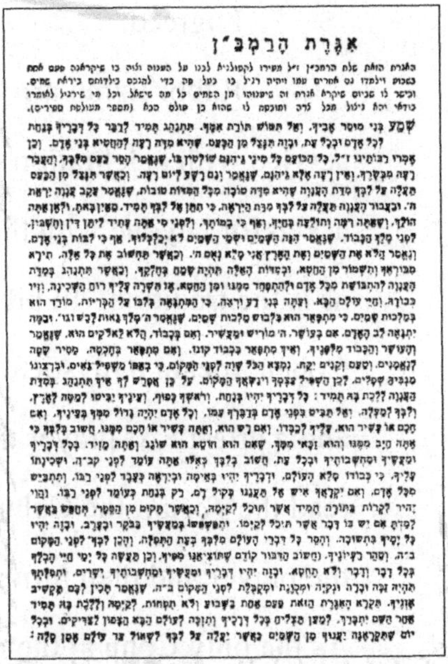
אגרת הרמב״ן

The first page of the Psalms was too small to read. According to Kabbalistic tradition, one should sit in the synagogue the entire night and read the Psalms of King David, Tikkun Olam, and the Talmud.

Background Landmark Synagogue

Richmond District, 4th ave SF CA

I agreed.

Rabbi Ezran arrived, and we began the *Shacharit* service with celebration of the *Torah.* Rabbi Ezran then asked for anyone with the surname Cohn to bless the *Torah*, as is the tradition. In biblical times the surname Cohn, or Cohen, meant a mystical healer. It also signified a leader and a priest. At prayer time, before opening the Ark to read the *Torah*, the Cohn would stand facing the Ark for the prayer and then turn around and bless the congregation. As the only Cohn at the morning prayer service, I began reading the *Torah.*

I was stunned. The section I was asked to read was about Moses receiving the Ten Commandments on Mount Sinai over three thousand years ago. In my dream, Moses had commanded me to make healing my life's mission and purpose. It was then that I fully realized the importance of my dream about Moses. It was significant that this dream came at the time of *Shavuot*, a holiday beginning the harvest. Gradually, I began to understand the "conclusion." I was being "commanded" to "harvest" my gift of VQH and produce "fruits" in the form of healed persons. Yet at this moment I still considered myself completely unqualified. If this experience is not a miracle, I don't know what is!

36. The Impact of Rabbi Shimon Bar-Yochaii

Three weeks later, Rabbi Shimon Bar-Yochaii appeared to me in a dream. According to Nobel Laureate Elie Wiesel in his book *Souls on Fire,* Rabbi Shimon Bar-Yochaii lived in the second century A.D. He was the famous master whose teachings are frequently quoted

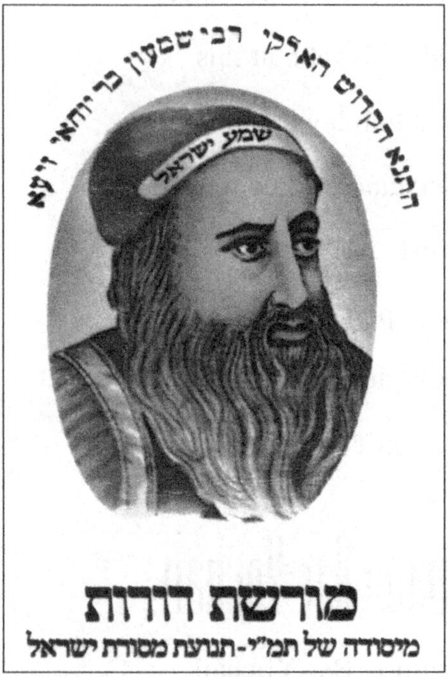

Rabbi Shimon Bar-Yochaii

The famous master whose teachings are frequently quoted and expounded in the Talmud. According to tradition, he is the author of the Zohar, the central Kabbalistic text, a mystical commentary on the Torah.

and expounded in the *Talmud.* He was condemned to death for having criticized the Roman occupiers, but he succeeded in escaping.

Along with his son, Elazar, the Rabbi took shelter in a cave where he spent thirteen years. There are numerous legends woven around this period in his life. It was said that he explored the mysteries of the *Kabbalah* during his seclusion and laid the foundation for the *Zohar, The Book of Splendor*. The *Zohar* is the central work of the *Kabbalah.* It offers a mystical commentary on the *Pentateuch* and its authorship is traditionally attributed to Rabbi Shimon Bar-Yochaii.

Later in my dream, the Rabbi was standing beside the *Torah* and *Zohar* in the cave of Meron near Safed, in the most northern part of Israel, in Galilee. As he left the cave, I ran after him and begged, "Rabbi — what should I do?"

"Take a seat inside with the other students and learn. That's all."

Later in my dream, I walked to a beautiful garden with enormous, colorful flowers, and saw something I had never seen before: very tall trees with unusual velvet flowers in a grassy meadow. There was no human presence to care for this extraordinary garden. Gorgeous peacocks, doves, and mythological animals including white unicorns, colorful pheonixes, exotic birds roamed freely, but there were no humans. Far in the distance, I saw a person dressed in the white garb of a prince, with a huge aura around him.

It was the Buddha, sitting under a large tree. He was handsome, with long hair and liquid dark eyes. I approached and greeted him with the most gentle voice. He replied, "You look lost." I sat next to him and he took both of us flying into the ethereal heaven.

"We're not airplanes, are we?" I asked.

Pointing in every direction, he thundered, "There are signs everywhere to help you find your healer's path!"

I awoke somewhat confused. I know nothing about Buddhism and little of Eastern philosophy, yet it seemed that I was receiving direction from many different spiritual powers to become serious and begin my mission of Visionary Quantum Healing.

It became clear to me that I have been given a gift that is meant to be shared for the benefit of others. When I look back at my family lineage, it is apparent that this gift extends hundreds, if not thousands, of years into the past. So I am compelled to be a Visionary Quantum Healer by a sense of duty as well as by a Buddha-like compassion for suffering humanity.

By using VQH, I have been able to heal otherwise incurable health problems. Many times people come to me when they have exhausted all other forms of treatment—both conventional Western medicine and even holistic-based Eastern therapies.

Chapter Six More Healing Methods

37. Dr. Richard Bloom Demonstrates on Salomon Cohn

Early in 1998, I attended an American Council of Hypnotherapy Examiners (A.C.H.E.) conference in Los Angeles. I have always had my healing gift, but sometimes its power is overwhelming, causing me some hesitation and even trepidation. I have explored various modalities, not to search for healing power but to try to better understand, connect with, and utilize fully the gifts I already possess. I thought that perhaps under hypnosis, I could address my fear and at last connect with and fully unleash the power of Visionary Quantum Healing. The following is an example of hypnomeditation, which can be used by the reader to enhance his own healing power and as a tool to heal others. This technique is covered in more detail later in this chapter in the section on "Healing and Hypnomeditation."

The following excerpts are from my momentous meeting with Dr. Richard Bloom, Ph.D., C.H.T., and Director of the Santa Monica Hypnotherapy Center. He was conducting a seminar about hypnotherapeutic mind/body healing techniques; we had never met before he addressed this seminar. It was at Dr. Bloom's suggestion that I entered a state of hypnotherapeutic induction.

"Salomon, would you like to come up, please? Have a seat." Then he turned to the seminar audience.

"This is going to be a wonderful experience for me, for Salomon, and I hope for all of you. This is an example of somebody who just walks in and says, 'What can you do for me?' You know what to do, and then you do it. Now, I need to tell you how this came about. What's nice about all of this is that I don't really know anything about Salomon. We haven't done an intake or anything else. During lunch today, Salomon said to me, 'Dr. Bloom, perhaps you can help me.' 'Perhaps,' I said. As Salomon talked, it occurred to me that he might consider doing a session during the symposium. Salomon consented, and here we are."

Dr. Bloom continued, "In the course of our conversation, Salomon mentioned that he does two kinds of healing. One is a natural air, light, and healing energy in which he uses a process he has developed. The other involves transmitting energy through his hands. They are both very powerful procedures. He is not asking me to help him get his power back. Rather, he wants to know, how can he integrate and double his power? Somehow, he is unable to use natural air, light, and healing energy and hand healing power at the same time. That is his problem. While Salomon and another guest were talking at the table, I suddenly got it. So with your permission, I am going to do the best I can."

Besides demonstrating the importance of improvisation, the session with Dr. Bloom showed that my two healing methods could be integrated. But the discovery of their potential to work as a single form of healing was made possible by my willingness to explore my own potential and move beyond my own self-perceived limits as a healer.

Dr. Bloom continued with the demonstration,

emphasizing his reliance on intuition and instinct:

Salomon, are you ready? Take a deep breath and hold it for two seconds. As you begin to exhale, slowly let your eyes close until I tell you to open them. Allow yourself to go deep. Take another deep breath; hold it for two seconds and exhale – slowly. Each time you exhale, go deeper and deeper and deeper. Good.

Now take a third deep breath. As you exhale slowly, feel that every cell in your body and mind is becoming completely relaxed. It feels as if this entire experience was meant to be. Beginning with coming here, my talking, your talking – all leading up to now. We both knew this is where we were going to end up – didn't we?

Addressing the audience, Dr. Bloom affirmed my gifts: "I have told Salomon that he possesses rare gifts, some of which are frightening to him." Turning to me, he said: "They are so unusual that they scare you."

Dr. Bloom spoke softly as he continued, *You will have to get past a lot of stuff just to get used to counting from one to ten, and I want your combined healing energy to grow stronger and stronger, until when I say the word 'ten,' it will be at full force.*

One, two, three – bring the healing energy up to the surface. Four, five, six – stronger and stronger, not using it, just having it there. Seven, eight, nine – there you will see a slot that says, Natural Air, Light, and Healing Energy. And ten – just park the healing energy in that slot.

Next to that slot is another that says, Hand Healing Energy. I now want you to focus on that as I count from one to ten and bring the hand healing energy up until it is in its slot.

One, two, three — think about the miraculous healing power of your hands. Four, five, six — coming up stronger and stronger.

Seven, eight, nine, ten, and put the hand healing energy there, right next to the air, light, and healing energy. If both of those healing energies are in place right next to each other, raise your first finger upward to indicate 'yes.' Good.

Now I want you to create an opening in the innermost part of your subconscious and your soul. I want you to create an opening through which the energy of both these healing powers can flow. As soon as you have done this, raise your first index finger upward, and this will indicate 'yes.' Good.

Now I am going to count down from ten to one. As I do, the energy of both powers, the hand power and the mind power, will combine and flow into this opening. When I reach zero, they will be combined inside you, forever.

Ten, nine, eight — feel those energies flowing, getting smaller and smaller as they flow into the opening. Seven, six, five—flowing more and more. Feel the power, the potential of your healing, doubling as it happens.

Four, three — it's incredible. This has never happened to you before, but the healing energy all seems to fit as if it belongs there. Two, one — Excellent!

Now I want you to imagine all the people in the world you have met and all of the people you have healed, and all the people in the world that you can now heal, because you have got double this power.

I want you to envision your family and friends and the people that you have healed and ask them for permission to combine your incredible powers to be even better than you are now. Ask for their approval. Let me know if anyone says 'no.' If they all approve, indicate 'yes.' They do? Everyone says, 'Yes!' In fact, they insist on it, don't they?

Now envision all the people you will heal — you won't see their faces, but you will feel their auras. You are going to be able to heal them now. Ask them how much they want you to use this double power. Feel as if it's an obligation. You hardly have the right to say 'no.' You have to do this, don't you? Must do this.

I am going to count from one to ten, and when I reach the count of ten and touch your forehead, this will be permanently melded inside you. You will never, from this moment on, be unable to use both powers. You will be able to use your hand energy and your VQH at the same time.

One, two, three — it feels so comfortable with those two energies combined — four, five, six — completely logical, and now you understand why you came here, took this workshop, went to lunch with me. And I understand it, too.

Seven, eight, nine, ten — take a deep breath and feel how everything is much more comfortable. Because everything is in place, where it belongs. It feels completely organic. Very, very good.

I want to thank your subconscious for working with us. I want to thank the part of you that went through a great deal of emotion to do this. We had to break through an incredible amount of fear. There are probably half a dozen little Salomons screaming, 'What are you doing to me? I don't want to change. The last time I changed, I almost died.' The ego resists change and clings to familiarity because spiritual change or expansion transcends ego and your identity is threatened. However, you were able to break through this fear because it was time. Your subconscious, your inner soul, told you it was time. It was OK to do this.

I congratulate you, and I thank you for allowing me to facilitate this healing for you. And I look forward to seeing you save many people, with even more power than before. Thank you very much.

Salomon, from the very bottom of your heart, thank that inner part of your subconscious that made all of this possible. And promise that you will continue to heal at double strength from now on. I want to give you one post-hypnotic suggestion. As you pass Janet Parks going back to your seat, I want you to permanently heal her back—making it even better than before, and confirming the healing.

All of the suggestions that you accepted are already working. You have done incredibly well.

You are feeling refreshed, restored, reborn, rejuvenated and repackaged. You are full of vitality and incredible healing energy. Back to here and now. Eyes open. Take a deep breath and stretch.

This demonstration shows how healers can realize greater and greater potential, but only if they are on good terms with the different parts of the subconscious. Prior to this session, I was using just the touching energy of "laying on of hands." Or I was just bouncing natural air, light, and healing energy. Before they were merged, the parts were weaker and the practices less efficient; now, merged, two healing energies can deliver more than double the power. However, touching was left behind because it was no longer necessary. Indeed, the new approach was different and more powerful, working on the physical and emotional planes. Moreover, an approach that is non-invasive and does not require disrobing has an additional legal benefit, since only physicians may legally use touch when healing.

Visionary Quantum healers must be able and willing to allow a method such as hypnosis to operate on the subtle levels of the psyche. I possess not only the gift of healing but also the capacity to work in tandem with another healer to develop his gift. The benefits of Dr. Bloom's hypnotherapeutic session are further described below.

38. Instant Cure for Janet Parks.

After leaving the stage, I immediately looked for Janet Parks. She is the woman Dr. Bloom suggested I heal when I awoke from my hypnotic state.

I found Janet in the middle of the audience. I asked her to go on stage with me for a healing treatment, and she agreed. On stage, Janet and I stood facing each other, about five feet apart. I asked her to allow her legs to be the sole support of her body, and to close her eyes and not open them until told to. I then asked her to feel her suffering and to rate the depth of that pain from zero to ten. Janet responded with a number less than ten and I asked her to amplify the pain as much as possible so that she could easily connect with it. By amplifying her pain, Janet could feel the changes and relief more immediately and dramatically. Janet's eyes remained closed, and I began transmitting a laser-like beam of natural air, light, and healing energy, inundating her with the full force of healing. Her aura became intensely vibrant.

While I gave Janet the treatment on stage, Dr. Bloom whispered to the audience, "Salomon is working on her now. He is channeling his energy and vision through his hands to Janet. Her body is shaking. She is visibly affected."

I gradually moved my hands higher, cleansing one chakra at a time, doing three repetitions on each. With full force, I bounced the beam of natural air, light, and healing energy back and forth over her face and ears. Moving from the lower torso upward, my hands generated beams of natural air, light, and healing energy that engulfed her shoulders and spine. In this way I purged the internal and external foreign entities, diseases that dispersed completely, vanishing out of the crown chakra. When I was finished, I told Janet, "You may open your eyes." I then cut the imaginary invisible rope around my neck and waist and moved away.

Janet was crying. "Incredible!" Dr. Bloom said. "Janet, come here. You may hug Salomon first. Can you talk? I'm sorry, but I need to get this right if we can. What happened?"

Still crying, Janet answered, "I don't know what happened!"

"What did you feel?"

"It was like all of the fears, the pain, everything was scrambling for its existence. It felt like there were energy charges going through my body. There aren't words to explain it."

"What we saw when Salomon extended his hands," Dr. Bloom explained to Janet, "is that you got from him a perfect healing energy. He was using his hands and vision. Your entire body was shaking!"

"I'm still shaking!," she exclaimed, laughing. "And my back does not hurt! Look, Dr. Bloom." Janet bent side to side, arched her back and then leaned forward. "I can move in any direction without pain."

"When Salomon went around to your back," Dr. Bloom continued, "you shook from another direction. You were crying. And now I can see that when you do work of this kind, it's so emotional that it's difficult to get people to talk about it immediately. But it was wonderful! Thank you very much."

By healing Janet's back, I discovered that my new powers were complete.

Some months after this event I received the following letter and release from Janet.

Testimonial

4/19/98

Dear Solomon,

You treated me for a condition I've had since 1986 at the ACHE Conference a couple of months ago.

I'm pleased to say that, other than what may have been one recurrence I have been symptom-free since February. I can't tell you what a relief it is to be symptom-free! It's been a <u>long</u> time.

Thank you so much. I've already begun telling others about you. My best wishes to you as you continue your good work.

Sincerely,

J. Parks, CHT, M.A.

39. Natural Light: Healing Energy Empowerment

During my hypnotic induction with Dr. Bloom, I had powerful visions of both those begging me to begin healing and those who would want to be healed. In the post-hypnotic session, I realized that this awesome power was frightening. I was not even sure where I was. When I healed Janet — it seemed so natural and fast — even I was amazed. Yet I was still filled with trepidation.

I got up from the chair after the hypnotic session with Dr. Bloom, and felt hands hovering over my shoulders. The hands were filled with enormous power - full of pure light healing energy. I "saw" my mother's grandfather, my great-grandfather, Rabbi Chaiim Pinto. He had a grand white beard, was dressed in gold and white cloth, and was engulfed in intense light energy. He goaded me, "Go and heal. Heal, heal!" The intensity overwhelmed me. Suddenly I felt empowered with natural light healing energy. I felt like light itself. I stood up and looked around, but could only see light as if I were living in the sun!

I saw myself garbed in white robes, near a small farmhouse atop a hill, in the midst of a multitude. Some people were healed and ecstatic; others were praying, waiting to be healed. My family was in joyous celebration. As the vision

תמונת הרב הקדוש מגא דמשפטים כמוהר״ר חיים פינטו זלה״ה זיע״א

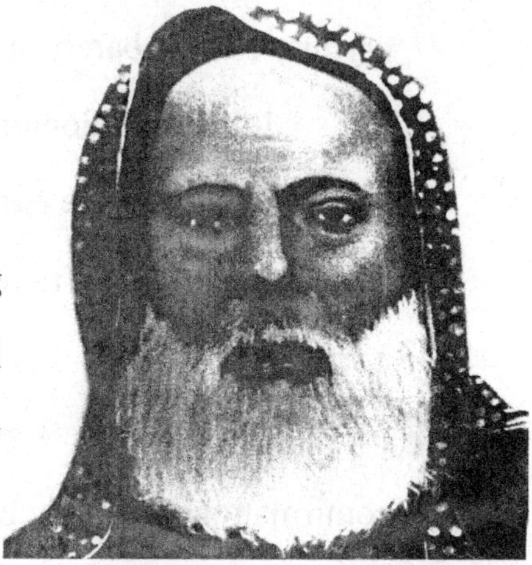

Rabbi Chaiim Pinto

Unable to reckon with the
awesome power I possessed,
I quit for many years. Then
prophetic visions started
coming to me—
Moses,
Rabbi Chaiim Pinto,
Rabbi Shimon Bar-Yochaii,
the Buddha—
All pushing me—
"Go and heal!"

vanished, I found myself in the post-hypnotic session, crying. I could barely speak.

In the tradition of others who have heard a higher calling, I have experienced doubt, deemed myself unworthy, and felt afraid of my powers. Just as healing is a relational practice focusing on the shared energy of the universe, trust in one's gift often requires the support and confirmation of close relatives and friends. The power to heal is larger than the person who is its conduit. Working with Dr. Bloom helped me realize even greater powers, while bringing me into spiritual contact with others.

This is a long process, but one that other healers can pursue. While the hypnosis was, for me, pivotal and dramatically transformative, the longer process of coming to grips with my new powers was ultimately decisive.

40. Awesome Healing Power

Before leaving the stage I told the audience, "I would like to relate one story to you. A dear friend of my wife's was scheduled for surgery for liver cancer. She and her husband joined us for dinner the night before she was to enter the hospital, and during the meal she complained of a headache. I suggested that she allow me to give her some healing energy. She was reluctant, but her husband assured her."

"When I started the treatment, she screamed."

"What's wrong?" her husband asked. "Salomon has hardly moved his hands."

"She explained that the moment my hand hovered over her head, she experienced enormous pain in the neck area. I continued working with her for fifteen minutes. The healing energy was becoming effective, and now she was comfortable."

"The reason I'm saying all of this is that she had been receiving treatment for cancer for the last two years. She was scheduled for surgery the next day. When she entered the hospital, she found out that her medical records had been misplaced. The clerks contacted other hospitals, but without success. The records had disappeared. Irate, she insisted upon being examined. The results came in, and the doctors said that she had no evidence of ever having had liver cancer. When I found out about this, it scared me. Unable to reckon with the awesome power I possessed, I quit practicing healing for many years, but dreams and visions soon started coming to me — Moses, Rabbi Shimon

Bar-Yochaii, Rabbi Chaiim Pinto, the Buddha - all pushing me to 'Go and heal!'"

Once again, my subconscious knew better than my conscious mind.

41. Healing and Hypno-Meditation

Hypno-meditation is a type of hypnosis that can be used on any client who wants to take advantage of this potent approach. A calm and pleasant natural environment will help the client to embrace the healing process. The hypno-meditative approach strengthens the client's entire body and can practically eliminate all diseases.

In working with these clients, I direct them as follows, drawing on my own experience with self-hypnosis:

"I urge you to remain fully conscious. Sit

comfortably and rest your arms softly, limply, at your sides. Let your eyelids close. Just relax every tiny muscle and nerve in and around your eyelids. Just relax, and go deeper. Now send a wave or beam of relaxation from the top of your head all the way, slowly, down to your toes. That will double the present level of relaxation. Now, with your body relaxed, I am going to help you relax your mind."

"Slowly you are slipping into a deep hypnotic sleep. Let us begin counting forward: one—close your eyes ... two—three... closed and heavy ... four ... five—closed and so sleepy ... six—sleepy ... seven—so very sleepy ... peaceful and relaxed ... eight—sleepy ... nine—so sleepy ... so sleepy ... ten—sleepy ... eleven—so completely and utterly relaxed ... feeling so peaceful and calm ... so free from tension...twelve—sleepy ... thirteen—drowsy and completely relaxed. Every muscle free from tension … fourteen. So sleepy … sleepy … fifteen—so sleepy … so sleepy … so … sleepy … so … sleepy. You are slipping into a deep, healing hypnotic sleep. You hear every word that I say … yet you are sound asleep … soundly relaxed and calm … and comfortable … very comfortable … you will continue to hear every word that I say."

"As you move from the trance to hypnotic meditation, you are imbibing the energy of nature. For a living organism and a human being, the most powerful substance on earth is the ozone (0_3), which is the master protector and the source of the energy being expressed. The ozone is the point of interface among all beings. The ozone allows for healing because, as a reactive antioxidant cleansing substance working with the trees and plants, it creates light rings of purity."

While the client is asleep, I continue to convey subliminally the following information to his or her subconscious: the ozone and the trees work together like different poles of an electric current, the same as Visionary Quantum Healing operates with natural air, light, and healing energy.

"As you and I accept healing," I continue, "trees, plants, and light rings of purity enter and surround our inner selves to protect us from harm at all times. These healing trees, plants, and light rings of purity symbolize the most powerful forces in all the universe. They protect us from all harm, from all invasions of bad entities, from negative outside influences and forms."

" Let's follow the process of healing through self-hypnosis. Allow yourself to think: a wall of protective and healing trees, plants, and light rings of purity is in and around me. It is my armor. I have learned to heal and love myself. And from this point on, as I repeat those words, I accept into my inner self the healing trees, plants, and light rings of purity in and around me for my protection. Transcendental protection of myself will spring into action, covering me with an armor of healing trees, plants, and light rings of purity, all of them healing."

Hypno-meditation involves covering ourselves with most powerful healing energy of trees, plants, and light rings of purity around us, embracing us wherever we go, so that we accept their healing into our inner selves. We are protected by nature itself. Trees, plants, and light rings of purity protect us. We are protected because the healing trees, plants, light rings of purity and our human being are one.

I now wake the client. " Now start counting to wake up. With each number you will begin to feel more alert and aware. Number one … Begin to awaken … Number two … Begin to wake up … Number Three … Eyes are opening … easily and gently …feeling invigorated … Number Four... Waking up... Move and stretch... Number Five... Waking up... Waking up."

Hypno-meditation is a useful alternative to VQH for trauma, chronic physical and emotional syndromes such as fear, phobias, degenerative disease, and pain relief. One or more sessions may be required, depending on the individual case. It can be done to oneself by recording the hypnotization from a practitioner or by recording one's own voice and playing it back.

42. The Dream of Human Limb Regeneration: 21st Century Healing

When Dr. Bloom asked me to envision all the people I would heal in the future, I saw thousands! I saw people suffering from all sorts of ailments, healed by me, as well as others empowered with the gift of VQH.

But the most astonishing, riveting image was that of an amputee whose limbs regenerated. I was awestruck! For many years, my most cherished dream has been to heal a person who has lost a limb. Deep inside, my gut feeling is that it can be done just by infusing mind power plus natural air, light, and healing energy. The starfish repairs and regenerates itself, as do the salamander and the earthworm. God willing, I believe that in my lifetime, I will be able to achieve this miracle.

The dream points to the infinite potential of VQH and the body's capacity to heal itself with light energy, and also sheds light on the healer's calling. The subconscious speaks to the healer in the language of dreams; the healer must trust in and listen to them. But a calling is mere potential without a method and a system to support that calling. The theoretical system that supports VQH is the Seven Major Chakras, described on pages 81-87.

43. Method: Treating Fertility Problems

In this instance, contrary to my usual practice, I do feel it is necessary to touch the client. When a practitioner must lay hands on a client, it is imperative that the client sign a release form. VQH practitioners must remember that they are not medical physicians. For more on this, see the section on "Healing and the Law" (p. 242).

However, the healing does not come from touch alone. To do this process, it is better for the client to sit or lie down, preferably the latter, since the position is more relaxed. The practitioner then lays one hand on the client's lower back, and the other hand on the woman's abdomen, next to the pelvis. Now the practitioner warms her ovaries by applying pure heat and light energy for about 15 minutes. The practitioner can converse with the client so that both will be at ease, and then both can relax for a few minutes. The practitioner then follows with the Four Phases of Visionary Quantum Healing (see pp. 109-134). Usually it only takes one session. Most clients achieve fertilization within a month. In rare instances, more sessions may be needed, at one-month intervals.

The following story describes my experiences using these fertility techniques. In 1970 I returned to Israel to visit my parents, friends, and family. At the home of one of my dear childhood friends, I asked, "How are your wife and children?" Daniel said, "Although we have been married for so many years, and have tried for the past seven years, my wife is unable to conceive. We have been seeing many doctors, but they cannot help us."

I told him that I could help.

With my friend and my sister present, I applied Visionary Quantum Healing to his wife. Then I instructed the couple to shower and make love, and my sister and I left.

A week later, I returned to the U.S. Three months later, my sister called me: "Tina's pregnant! She's going to have twins." Today Tina's healthy sons have completed high school and are serving in the Israeli military.

It happens again and again. The latest person is my niece Tami. After a splendid dinner at her house, she grabbed me and said, "Please Uncle, I want you to warm my stomach. I want to have one more baby!" I gave her one successful single treatment in front of the whole family. Nine months later, she gave birth to another girl: Uval.

44. Headache and Pain Elimination

Even though headaches can be healed with VQH, I have discovered another approach that is more direct and equally effective. It will eliminate headache and pain for good. I know, because I have had great success with hundreds of clients since the early 1970s by using this procedure. It is not necessary to have a headache, by the way, at the time that you have an appointment with the healer.

The client relaxes in a seat in front of the healer with his or her eyes closed throughout the entire session. Then the healer asks the client for the location of the headache and pain.

Q. "Where is your headache?"

A. "Right side."

Q. "If it had a weight, how heavy would it be ?"

A. "About one pound."

Q. "If it had a shape, what would it be ? Like a square ? Triangle ? Round or oval?"

A. "Round."

Q. "If it had a color, what would it be?"

A. "Black."

Repeat this questioning process at least three or four times. As you repeat the process, make sure to change the questions around. Make sure to communicate that foreign entities have no place in humans—that's why the headache's size, shape, or color keep changing. The dramatic changes in the headache's appearance establish that its causal agents are extrinsic to the person's healthy energy fields.

In the event that the headache has not been eliminated, repeat the process twice more, only this time have the client deeply inhale, then exhale to purge himself of the disease entities.

If you do the procedure correctly, you will eliminate the intensity and discomfort. The chances are good for both immediate and permanent success.

It is imperative when doing this process that you recall the patient's answers regarding previous locations, sizes, shapes, and colors.

45. Absentee Visionary Quantum Healing Treatment

VQH can be done from a distance. I use the following protocol to do a full body treatment:

A. Set a treatment time with the client. Ask him or her to lie down and relax during that period.

B. Imagine your client the size of a baby. If you have difficulty visualizing this, you may work with an actual teddy bear or doll, or you can work with a recent photo. Imagine your client being one with the doll or image.

C. Call on the healing guide, who is the higher self of the client. Also call on your own higher self to assist you in facilitating this treatment.

D. Draw the VQH energy over the client's symptom. Do a healing treatment. Research indicates it is best to start the treatment from the head down.

E. Ask that the VQH energy flow through you at the highest possible level that is beneficial for you and your client. Say the client's name during the treatment.

F. Send a thought to the client's being that it is his or her responsibility to take in the healing energy and use it to restore every cell to its anatomically perfect state.

G. If you are working with a teddy bear or doll, place one hand over its head, and the other hand over the symptom, throughout the entire healing.

H. If you are working with a photo, hold it with both hands to make a kind of "hand sandwich." (A healing can also be done on an animal by using a photo of that animal.)

Hypnosis of an exotic bird

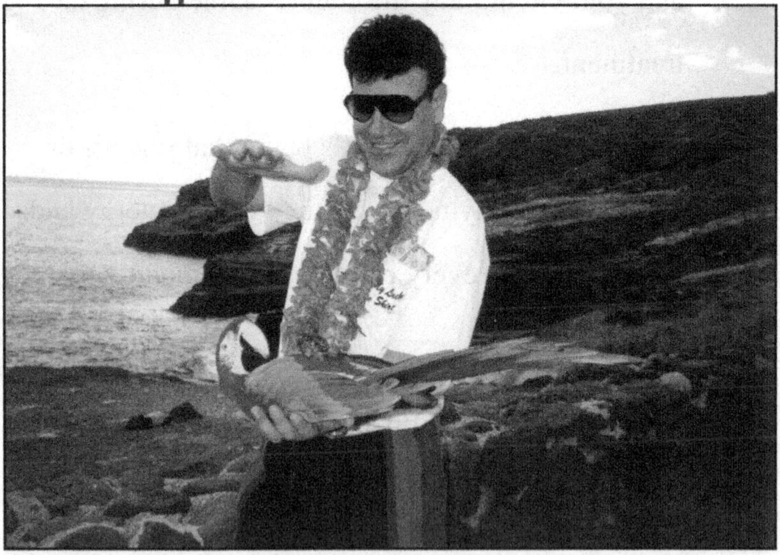

On the island of Hawaii, Dr. Salomon Cohn demonstrates the skill of hypnosis on an exotic bird.

I. When you are done, send the client's being back to him or her.

J. Then say, "I ask that your being easily and effortlessly integrate into your physical body."

After the absentee healing, keep the following in mind:

A. Research studies show that the treatment works best if the client is consciously aware that he or she is receiving a treatment, and can sit or lie down during the forty-five minutes to one hour session. It takes three times as long to transfer energy over a long distance.

B. It is a wonderful experience to give a VQH treatment to your own inner child, or to an image of yourself from a challenging year in your life.

C. If you use a photo, teddy bear, or doll, you can give the item to the client afterwards; it will continue to radiate VQH energy.

D. Except for soft music, there should be no background noise, especially television.

46. Psychic Coincidences

Telling Coincidences and Fond Recollections Following My Mother's Death.

On April 25, 2003, my Mom died at the age of 95 in Jerusalem, Israel. My sister Rachel, who lives in Jerusalem not far from where my Mother lived, called to notify me and my brother Oury at our homes in the United States. As sad as my brother was about our Mother's death, about an hour later he had an intuition that he should call his colleague David and tell him to stop praying for our Mom. Since Mother had been ill for the year prior to her death, my brother Oury had asked David, who had renewed his faith in religion, to pray at the synagogue often for Mother.

As soon as David heard Oury's voice, he interrupted, "I know why you're calling me … your Mom died." My brother was so stunned, he could barely speak. His intuition to call David was right.

"How do you know?" Oury asked. "My sister just called me from Jerusalem and told me so. There's no way in the world you could have known."

David replied, "No, you don't understand — I mean that I was just about to call you too. You see, your Mom appeared in my dream as beautiful, strong and righteous, with a white aura all around her. My dream was so vivid that I awoke shaken. She told me that she was going away and she asked me not to pray for her any more! From now on she will pray for my children and me. Oury, yes, your Mom is righteous."

"I thank you, David, for praying for my Mom," Oury said.

"No," David replied, "thank you for granting me this great privilege. Shabbat Shalom."

I found myself wondering if we had inherited this psychic ability from our dear Mom. This personal anecdote underscores for me the reality of parapsychological and spiritual phenomena, and thus supports the credibility of non-Western healing practices.

Chapter Seven A Final Note

47. A Near-Death Experience Occasions Great Discovery

On July 14, 1998, my children Ari and Ilana, and their friend Lisa visited me in San Francisco. We planned to spend a wonderful week together. I am a certified free-fall skydiver and invited everyone to go skydiving with me. They took an intensive "crash" course and we went skydiving at nearby Davis the next day. We put on the chutes before walking to the plane. As a certified teacher of tarot, palmistry, and matters metaphysical, I read everyone's hand. "OK," I said to the kids, "safe journey to all."

My son Ari said, "Since you have read our palms, how about yours?"

"If you insist." On my hand a big square appeared on my lifeline, showing the exact time that indicated my current age. I was both dismayed and astonished, and the look on my face conveyed these emotions.

"Tell us what you see, Dad."

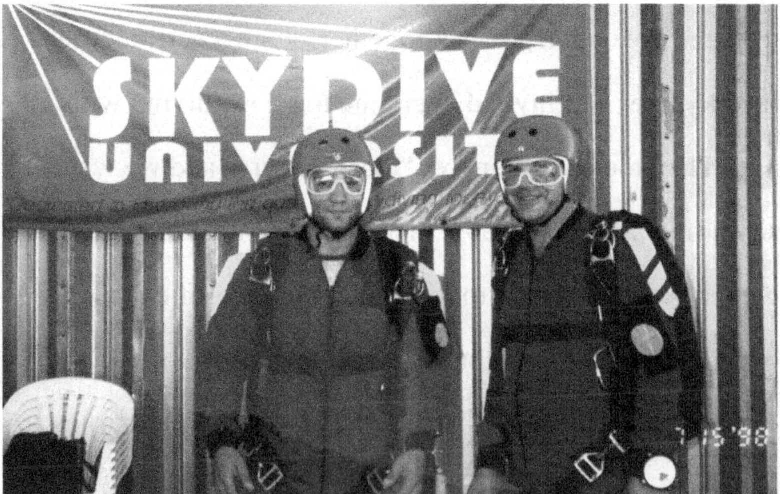

My son Ari and me

"Up In The Sky I Am The 'Master' Of My Domain"

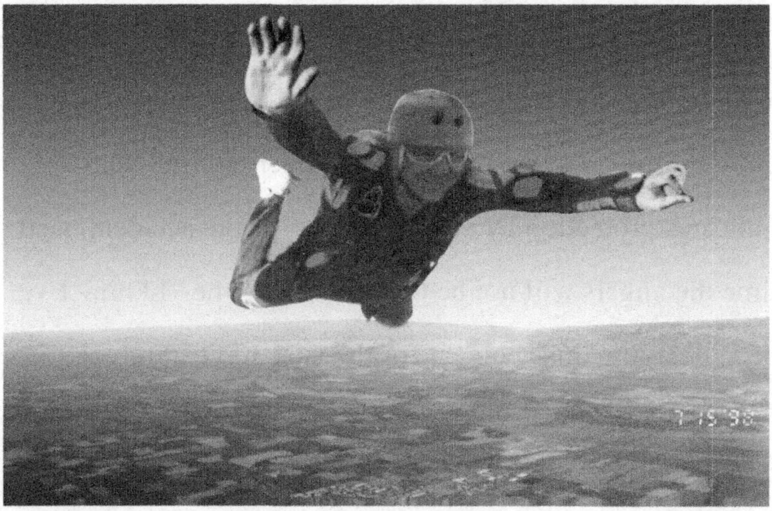

Salomon's last free fall from 9500 feet

I replied, "I'll be OK."

"What do you mean?"

I showed him my hand and explained the lines.

"You see, I will parachute with you guys and most likely I

will be injured. It is inevitable. However, angels will be looking over me."

This answer really angered Ari. "You're sick, Dad! Why parachute if you know you're going to be injured?"

"Ari," I replied, "the square over my lifeline indicates protection by angels. If I delay the accident, next time the angels will not be there to rescue me. I know I've been delaying this accident for the past 30 years, since I first learned palmistry."

We boarded the plane and soared into the sky.

48. Free Fall and Out-of-Body Experience

When we reached altitude, one by one, we jumped and did a free fall from nine thousand, five hundred feet. In the final five hundred feet, we planned to open our chutes, making a turn. At about six stories above the ground, however, the inevitable did happen — the wind caught my ropes and wrapped them around the chute. There was no time to open the spare chute. I landed very hard on the ground and died for a minute or so.

Then a transformative out-of-body experience ensued. I thought, "That's it." Suddenly I was guided by a being of light, sucked into a void through a white tunnel. At the far end of the tunnel, people were shouting, "Go back! Go back, you have work to do!" My sky diving accident had nearly ended my life: but I was saved by angels!

Just before I opened my eyes, two angels hovered over me, telepathically communicating with me: "You're protected, Salomon. Just breathe. Open your eyes."

Then I recall someone pumping my heart and yelling, "Welcome back!" I heard his words while I was still motionless. "What is your name? Do you know where you are?" He was a paramedic, shouting questions at me while he cut off my jump suit. When the paramedics moved me to the gurney and strapped me down, the pain began — awesome pain. I kept demanding a painkiller. The paramedic gave me a shot, probably of morphine.

The next thing I knew, I was in a helicopter on the way to the hospital. I had serious injuries: a liver laceration, a fractured rib, a spine with two-thirds of the vertebrae fractured, a fractured arm, a fractured leg, and a fractured shoulder. Dr. Mark Field and Dr. Steven Goldberg told me, my family, and my colleagues (Paul Rosen, Ph.D., and David Webster, M.D.) the bad news: I would never walk again.

With what little voice I had, I said that they should not bet on it. I would walk in no time.

Palm Reading of Being Saved By Angels

Box feature over lifeline at the time of accident on Salomon's hand indicating protection of angels

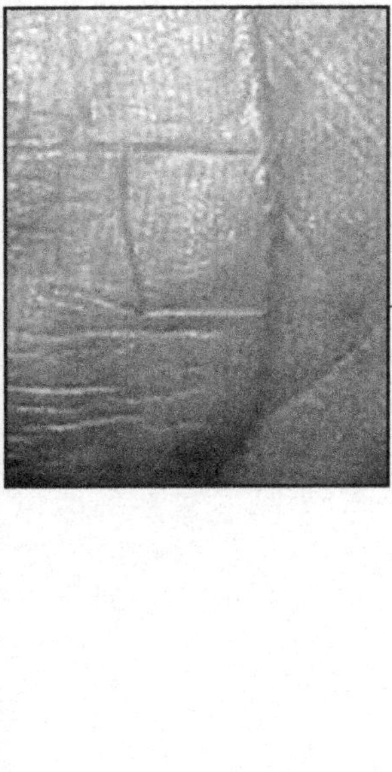

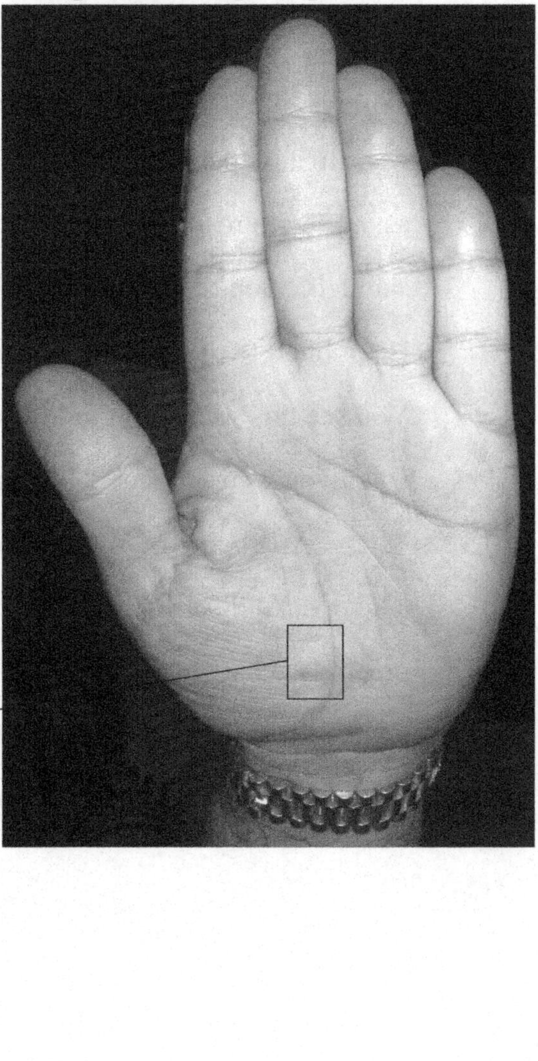

49. Confirmation of Being Saved By Angels

Two days later my children, Ari and Ilana, came to visit me in the hospital. Jay, my metaphysics professor, was already there. I introduced everyone. My children asked Jay to read my palm. After one quick glance, Jay shouted, "Son of a gun! You have been saved by angels!" He pointed to the lines on my hand. "Look at your lifeline. You see this square? It indicates a specific time of your life when you were protected by angels."

Ari shouted, "Wow! Dad told us so. Right before take off. And he insisted that he would be OK. He said precisely what you have said — that he would be saved by angels, and that this was probably the only time that the angels would be there. Frankly speaking, I was a bit skeptical."

Because of my out-of-body experience, I am certain that we can know about death. But there is so much more to learn; it is far greater than what we think we know. My path toward after-life experience became clear! It propelled my destiny and revealed to me the meaning of life.

But in the meantime, I faced the daunting prospect of healing.

50. From Agony to Ecstasy: Moments of Discovery

In physical shock from my injuries, and in psychic shock from the out-of-body experience, the intervention of the angels, and the medical reports, I had never been so down.

I had serious physical injuries. At first I followed the medical paths laid out by the doctors at UC Davis Hospital, including traction but no casts, along with guidelines from my own training as a healer and clinical hypnotherapist. I worked hard in physical therapy for the next two months, but saw myself making little real progress. I drew upon my knowledge of self-hypnosis, but this practice provided only minor relief, not a cure. Out of discouragement, and prompted by my interest in nature, I sought to be my own version of a true healer.

This led to the discovery of the three key elements of Visionary Quantum Healing. As I lay in the hospital bed and gazed out the window at the trees, I began to imagine a mode of healing based on incorporating natural energy flow. These trees, and by extension other green plants, all require light. It occurred to me that the self-hypnosis

I had studied could be evolved to feature the energy and the purity of light. To this mix I added the Hebrew idea that air, spirit, and healing are one. I realized that healing involves natural air, light, and healing energy.

Soon after, I stopped taking medication and avoided having any kind of surgery. In order to somehow transcend my physical, mental, and spiritual trauma, I journeyed back, using self-hypnotic meditation, to my condition prior to the accident. I embraced images of plants and trees, bringing them within me to create the light rings of purity. Increasingly, scientific research shows that exposure to nature, such as looking at trees from a hospital room window, contributes significantly to health and healing. My healing was not instantaneous, but it did, over time, work wonders. (See p. 181 for my discussion of hypno-meditation.)

51. The Attentive Angel of Love

When I was a young boy, an economic recession during the 1950s cost my Dad his job as an electrical engineer. While he was out of work for a full year, my mother, who was a middle-school teacher, became the sole support for our family. She still found time to take care of a family of seven young children, keeping us neat and aware of important values such as education. Despite the small income she received, delicious food was always prepared and set attractively on the table. To this day, I wonder how she ever managed to support our family with such gracious simplicity.

I also recall once when, as a boy of nine, my younger brother Oury was sick with a high fever. While Mom was attending to his well-being, I asked her whom she loved the most. She answered with her special gaze.

Whether her big hazel eyes were downcast or smiling, we knew exactly what she was feeling. It's amazing how well she trained us to read the meaning in her look and her facial expression, without saying a single word. I guess this non-verbal communication is something that we grow up and learn how to live with (out of respect and love). Yes, she applied her special magic to our home life.

In addition to her ability to communicate non-verbally, Mom was also skillful with words. Pointing to my sick baby brother, she responded, "Right now your brother needs me; you and your siblings can take care of yourselves. I love you, too. Now do your homework and off you go." At an early age I learned the crucial importance of verbal and non-verbal communication, as well as nurturing love. I applied this experience in later years in developing alternative methods of healing.

52. The Link to Salomon through Past Lives

I was born with the gift of healing. My mother, through her dreams about her grandfather, Rabbi Chaiim Pinto, made a connection between my name and healing. Like me, the biblical Salomon was a magician. In the mystical book *Clavicula Salomonis*, he is described as possessing the key to healing. Although I have over forty certifications, including Clinical Hypnotherapy, Reiki, Reflexology, and Inner Massage Therapy, family inheritance also possesses the gift of healing. Healing is in both my nurture and my nature.

During my past life regression, conducted by Dr. Jean Schurz, Ph.D., Director of the Inner Quest Awareness Institute of California, she exclaimed, "You were King Salomon and later, another great healer in ancient Israel,

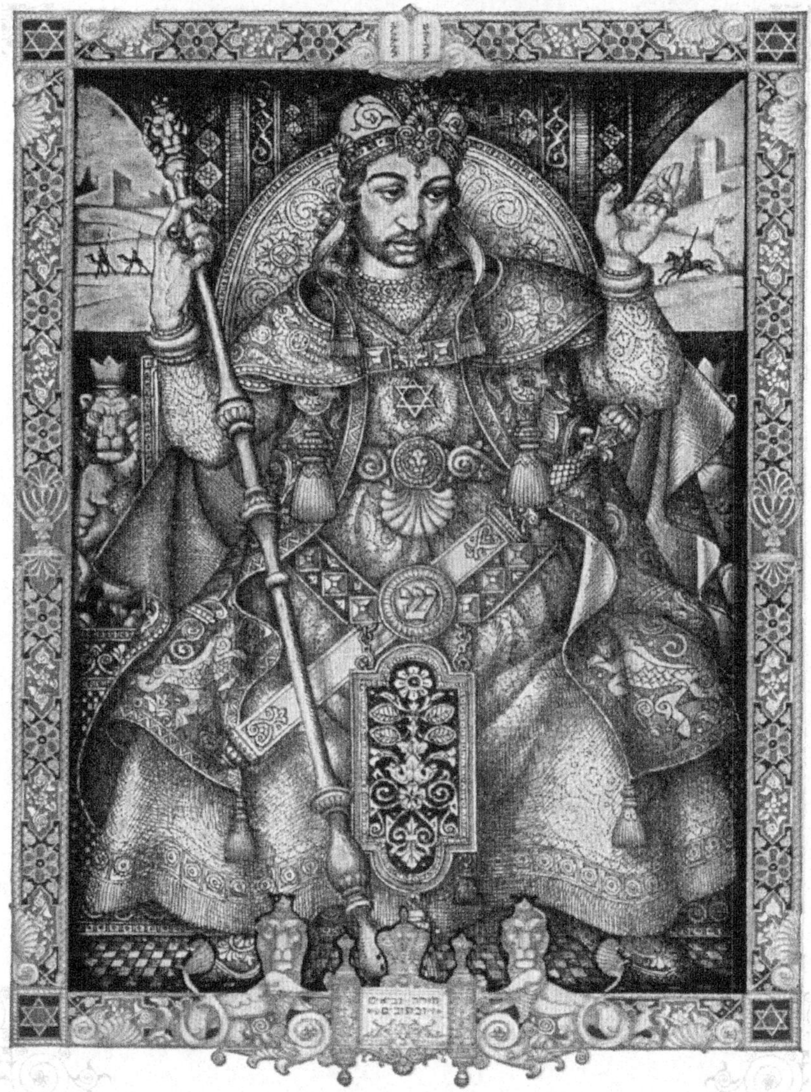

Salomon the Wise
"Happy is the man who finds wisdom..."

with numerous followers in northern Galilee in ancient Israel about 100 B.C. You were a trusted advisor and lover of Queen Isabella of Spain at the end of the fifteenth century."

I do remember being Queen Isabella's advisor and lover. When this situation was discovered, the Queen's husband, King Ferdinand, tried to hang me without a trial. Of course, I tried to escape.

I awoke from the regression crying. The trance had vanished.

Later, Dr. Schurz again induced a hypnotic trance to allow me to return to the past. I was trying to reach my earlier past as King Salomon the Healer — but it was impossible. I did, however, go back to Spain as Queen Isabella's advisor. Again, King Ferdinand tried to hang me, and again, I awoke in tears.

My healing gift has traveled with me through the ages. As Einstein showed us, time does not travel ceaselessly in one direction; it is relative, and can be transcended. I was, am, and will be a healer.

53 How VQH Differs From Well-known "Medical" Healing Techniques

Visionary Quantum Healing is more than a healing process. While I was developing VQH, I found that it works a lot faster with natural air, light, and healing energy. I realized this healing awakening would take you down to the path of the self-healing. As a student and practitioner of VQH, the process will teach you how to visualize and see the unseen. VQH is a glimpse into the depths of the human experience.

To take a look at this point, consider the life force of breathing. The VQH process works quite naturally throughout the body, with clothes on or off. This is the reason that the body is breathing natural air, light, and healing energy at all times with the assistance of the practitioner.

Looking for the ultimate cure, here is the irony. In my academic career, I researched healing in ancient and contemporary cultures. In fact, I have been on a healing quest for the past three and half decades. Over the course of this quest, I performed thousands of successful healing treatments.

On December 1, 2005, CNN evening news anchor Anderson Cooper was discussing the alternative views on healing presented by representatives of Scientology and psychiatry. Bruce Wiseman, President of the Citizens Commission on Human Rights and a member of the Church of Scientology, stated that psychiatry is a travesty and a crime, and damages the patient's brain with chemically induced imbalances. The Vice President of the American Psychiatric Association, Dr. Nada Stotland, emphatically denied any comparison between Scientology, a religion lacking any scientific proof or validity, and clinical psychiatry, an accepted field of science with extensive objective research. Dr. Stotland also commented that she did not agree to appear on the television broadcast to debate the merits of Scientology, which she said is based on pretext. She strongly defended psychiatry by comparing it to medical surgery as a legitimate field of modern medicine, citing brain imagery as objective evidence of its validity.

Cooper continued the broadcast by showing excerpts of video clips featuring the actor Tom Cruise on a recent Barbara Walters talk show about Scientology.

Cruise suggested that there is factual proof that Scientology has more of a basis in fact than psychiatry. Again, Scientologist Bruce Wiseman insisted that psychiatry is a pseudoscience, with psychiatrists pumping millions of patients full of mind altering drugs and subjecting 100,000 people to shock treatments each year.

These two opposing viewpoints are typical of the many belief system processes that are ineffective in treating cases of mental and physical disease.

In October, I was invited to a private party. After mingling with the other guests, the host introduced me to a group of five medical surgeons and their wives. They were all happily laughing, speaking loudly, and introducing themselves to each other by name. The rest of the group referred to each other as doctors or, more precisely, as butchers. I find their comments, as evidenced by the names they called each other, not surprising to me at all. I gazed at them with sadness and empathy because of the cynical way they made these comments. I had been told in my youth, "When you drink wine, the secret will spills out." I guess drinking was their aim!

In my opinion, these approaches to healing - conventional medicine, holistic medicine, aromatherapy, Chinese medicine, homeopathy, and Scientology – just treat the patient with symptomatic relief, while providing no lasting cure. In contrast, VQH does provide a lasting cure because of its use of natural air, light, and healing energy.

In conclusion, with great perseverance, we shall change our ways of thinking by looking at this new method of healing. I want to convey, and I call upon the science community and medical technicians to do more research on VQH and to adopt this new concept that eventually will lead to an easy, fast, and beneficial cure that is financially affordable to almost everyone.

VQH is the new future healing treatment process that gives instantaneous cure to most chronic diseases. Conventional medicine and holistic methods are not exclusively failures for not looking for cures. Looking only for relief, with a mission to concentrating on the sales of conventional drugs, and simultaneously promoting the righting of chemical imbalance with herbal remedies is tremendous business. But all these methods are taking the wrong approach. VQH is the process that achieves total success for the patient while having as its basis the right approach.

It is the VQH healer who demonstrates that healing doesn't always require words. The healer teaches us to not give up and to keep pursuing the real Visionary Quantum Healing process, heal humans along with all living creatures, and to keep reaching out, successfully connecting, until the patient is cured. The practitioner, by truly healing someone, can ease pain and suffering in ways that words cannot. Sometimes, neither person needs to speak for a win/win situation to happen that results in successful healing treatment. This dream of mine from decades ago, Visionary Quantum Healing, is the great hope of today and of the future.

54. Frequently Asked Questions about Visionary Quantum Healing

The following questions are more extensively answered in my seminar on Visionary Quantum Healing. Perhaps you are asking the same questions yourself. Please take a moment to review the answers here:

Do we really need VQH?

Unlike other approaches, the VQH system does not require the client to embrace any belief system, nor is it impeded by one. The effectiveness of the Ayurvedic healing system and traditional Chinese medicine, for example, depend on the client's holding certain beliefs about balance and spirit. Although concepts of balance and spirit are useful for diagnosis, VQH does not rely on them. Indeed, VQH does not require a formal diagnosis to produce consistently effective treatment, when delivered by an expert practitioner. Moreover, its results are immediate.

Why do we believe in the VQH process?

VQH is not a belief system. It is based on scientific research and study. The case studies and testimonials are a tribute to the success of Visionary Quantum Healing.

What does VQH mean to me?

VQH addresses the client's physical and emotional condition and successfully treats difficult cases, usually requiring only one treatment.

Who benefits from VQH?

Bypassing the usual limitations, VQH attacks the problem directly, on the most fundamental plane of human existence — the human energy field. In this way, the VQH approach does not work solely from holistic assumptions and avoids the fallacies of Western and Eastern dualisms, such as the mind/matter split. Through using these techniques, your healing success will be much more consistent, and predictable.

Your effectiveness in working with others will be dramatically increased, and your ability to empower yourself for optimal results will be increased. You will be able to generate empowering emotional states within yourself at will, eliminate any negative emotions or limiting decisions, identify and change limiting beliefs, and inspire yourself with a compelling future that will have a much better chance of coming true.

How is VQH applied?

Visionary Quantum Healing involves the

transference of natural air, light, and healing energy between the practitioner and the client. It is a non-medical, non-invasive approach and no disrobing is required.

How long does it take for VQH to have an effect?

Healing usually results, to a large degree, in instant improvement, with full healing occurring over a period of a few days. With conditions that have been present a long time, it may take several weeks until maximal benefits are achieved. Diseases that cannot be cured by this different process are extremely rare.

Is VQH safe?

There are no known directly harmful effects of healing. VQH will occasionally bring about releases of emotions that were buried in the unconscious mind, usually related to symptoms that motivated a person to seek treatment. The process may temporarily intensify pain or other symptoms that are being treated. These are viewed as positive signs, indicating releases of blocked biological energies. VQH may provide instant relief from symptoms or may bring about gradual improvement of many conditions.

VQH is often used as a complement to both conventional and non-traditional therapies. You must ask your medical doctor whether VQH can be used for your condition instead of conventional treatments. Do not stop conventional treatments without consulting your physician.

Who is qualified to be a Visionary Quantum healer?

VQH is a scientific process that anyone can learn. There are gifted natural healers who have very strong healing gifts, and they will readily become skillful VQH practitioners. There are healers who have extensive training and years of experience, but they may not be particularly potent or good healers.

Visionary Quantum practitioners may qualify and be certified during a one-day seminar. VQH is not a licensed profession, it is a certification. Many of the alternative healing schools and organizations have recommended Codes of Conduct and Standards for Practice. Adherence to these is a matter of individual responsibility. While it is definitely worthwhile asking whether a Visionary Quantum healer is a member in good standing of a healing organization, there is no guarantee that you will benefit from his or her treatments.

Many people are unaware that they have healing gifts. Many professional caregivers may find that their hands become warm when they are tending patients, or their patients may notice the warmth. A mother kissing away the hurt of a child may be a healer. Many people discover their healing gifts when they place a hand compassionately on someone in need of comfort and are told that this helped dramatically, such as in distinctly alleviating pain.

Where can I find a Visionary Quantum practitioner?

The best route is through recommendations from trusted friends and caregivers. You may also contact the Visionary Quantum Healing Research Network at www.drcohn.net.

How do I choose a good Visionary Quantum practitioner?

As mentioned above, VQH is a scientific process.

The delicate, nearly palpable interpersonal vibrational chemistry that exists between any two people is particularly relevant to healing interactions. Finding a Visionary Quantum healer with whom you will resonate positively is a lot like finding a good friend, a psychotherapist, or a physician with a good bedside manner. Recommendations from satisfied clients, especially if you know and trust them, are your best leads. Referrals from trusted caregivers are your next best lead. Even with an enthusiastic recommendation, however, there is no guarantee that you will get along with the healer just because another person found the practitioner to be good. So be patient, and plan to do some preliminary investigation and telephone interviews before you go for treatment.

My personal belief is that many symptoms and

illnesses develop out of tensions and disharmonies — either within us or between ourselves and our environment (relationships and living/work situations). A good healer is often also a good counselor.

A cautionary note: Visionary Quantum Healing results are instantaneous and safe. A certified Visionary Quantum healer will spend 15 to 20 minutes doing the process of healing with you. Beware of healers who pressure you and warn that unless you come back for their specific treatments, your condition will deteriorate or you will die. No healer can predict such things with certainty. Healers may sense whether their treatments are likely to be of help, but an ethical healer will present an educated opinion and leave it up to you to decide, just as a wise physician will do.

Can anyone learn VQH?

VQH is a scientific process that anyone can learn by studying *The Complete Guide to Visionary Quantum Healing* and by attending a Visionary Quantum Healing seminar. If you are motivated to learn the process, you can expect to achieve competency as a VQH practitioner.

Are there any theories to explain VQH?

There are conventional scientific theories that explain spiritual healing. Biological energies of healers interact with those of clients to bring about changes. Also, the intentions, wishes, meditations and prayers of healers can influence the consciousness of the client, bringing about changes that then eliminate the client's problems. Scientific research, as well as the Kabbalah, numerology and geometry contributed to my discovery of the VQH process.

Is there evidence that VQH is effective?

Surveys of clients in several countries who have tried various methods of alternative healing show a satisfaction rate of 73 percent to 91 percent. These include studies of both humans and animals. Clients who have tried the VQH process, however, express an overall satisfaction rating of 98 percent.

Healers make broad claims about the benefits of their treatments. There is a broad spectrum of anecdotal reports about different methods and the significant effects of healings. There is now reason to believe that many of these healing reports have substance. The *Complete Guide to Visionary Quantum Healing* will radically change your perceptions of the world and how you can relate to yourself, to other people, and to your environment.

Healers present an enormous spectrum of approaches that can bring about improvements in many conditions that do not respond to conventional medical care. Some healers treat through a laying-on of hands, with a light touch, or with hands held near to, but not touching, the person. Other healers use massage, acupuncture, herbs, hypnosis, Reiki and Ayurvedic methods. On rare occasions there are very rapid, even instantaneous, transformations from illness to health. More often, there is a gradual decrease in pain, improvement in the client's physical condition, diminished anxiety, and a more positive, brightened outlook.

Holistic healing has been used since the dawn of history. It is still found in many unbroken traditions of shamanic healing. A century of research in parapsychology has confirmed the existence of mind-to-mind communications (telepathy), mind-matter awareness (clairsentience), and the effects of mind on matter (psychokinesis). A vast body of research confirms the reports of many healers.

Clarification on the subjective nature of research shows that there is no "objective truth." Even the most reliable research is open to interpretation. If the mind can interact with both living and inanimate matter, then researchers can actually influence the outcome of their own experiments. This has far-reaching implications for health care, spiritual awareness, and the healing of our environment. Healing enhances personal spiritual awareness and a deep inner knowledge that you are part of a vast, loving universe. Healing knows no limits. We can learn to extend healing to our ailing societies and our shared planet.

Western society has neglected, and even forgotten, healing in its explorations of biochemical medicine. But during the last decade there has been a notable shift in conventional attitudes toward healers. Research shows that spiritual healing may be helpful in treating heart conditions, AIDS, hypertension, muscle fatigue, arthritis, depression, anxiety, and stress. Studies in other species demonstrate the effectiveness of spiritual healing on wounds, in slowing or halting the growth of cancer, in altering the growth of plants, bacteria, and yeasts, and in influencing cellular and DNA functions. Healers are now being invited to collaborate with doctors, often in hospital settings, and nurses and doctors are learning to develop and use their own healing gifts. Healing is an effective, safe, and cost-effective complement to most traditional treatments.

Do I have to have faith to be healed?

There is no research evidence to suggest that faith is required to be healed with VQH. Humans, animals, and plants have responded to VQH. However, if you believe that faith is an essential part of your personal healing, it may be important for you to explore this belief and come to peace with it.

55. Conclusion

While VQH emerges from a cluster of contemporary holistic outlooks, it is an alternative, non-holistic and non-conventional medical treatment based on scientific research. The client need not adopt any belief system to benefit from its remarkable cures. VQH relies on natural air, light, and healing energy to restore energy flow and eliminate all entities (diseases) from within the client's body, mind, and soul. Thus it addresses the physical and the emotional realms, is non-invasive, non-verbal, and requires no touching.

The procedures laid out in this book are easy for practitioners, clients and students to learn and use. This text will serve as a teaching manual for the Four

Phase process of Visionary Quantum Healing. The book also offers additional curative processes for headache elimination, personal injury, absentee healing, fertility problems, hypno-meditation. and frequently asked questions about VQH. In the pages that follow are client information forms, release and consent forms, contracts, a section on healing and the law, instructive case studies, professional and client testimonials, a White House Commission Final Report on Health and Alternative Medicine (March 2002), an index, a recommended book list, and other useful illustrations.

VQH works on animals and on any mammals. The good thing about treating mammals is that there is no placebo effect. There are absolutely no side-effects. There are only side benefits. Based on the revolutionary Four

Phases, Visionary Quantum Healing is the secret to life.

I am convinced that this original and revolutionary healing curative process will endure and be handed down from generation to generation. This is because it brings about intense, rapid and satisfactory healing. I have lost my life more than once and have been declared paralyzed from neck down. Today, I look and feel great, a living testimony to VQH. The holistic health care and medical communities will adopt the Visionary Quantum Healing process with its use of natural air, light, and healing energy. This VQH process will be my legacy.

How can I

best help you?

By being

Sincere

Aware

Caring

Thoughtful

Empathetic!

Appendix A:

56. Healing and the Law

As a professional Visionary Quantum Healing practitioner, it is important that you are familiar with local, state, and federal government laws regarding what you legally can and cannot do in a treatment session.

There are very specific laws in all countries. In the United States the law states that you must be a licensed physician, chiropractor, nurse, practitioner, physician's assistant, osteopath, naturopath, physical therapist or licensed massage therapist in order to touch another person's body.

If you are not certified in at least one of these categories, in some states in order to perform VQH professionally, you must be an ordained minister. Many churches allow healers to become ordained ministers; check your phone directory for local churches.

The Universal Life Church strongly believes in the rights of all people to practice their beliefs, regardless of what those beliefs are, as long as they do not infringe on the rights of others and are within the law. To become a minister, send a letter stating your desire to become an ordained minister (with or without a donation) and address it to:

Universal Life Church
601 3rd Street
Modesto, California 95351
Phone: 209-527-8111

You can also go to the website at www.ulc.org for more information and to become an ordained minister online.

Cohn - Visionary Quantum Healing™

The following forms are to protect every practitioner, holistic or conventional, by law, and also to protect the integrity of the profession.

57. Client Information

Last Name: ______________ First Name and Initial: ____________

Address: ____

Day Phone: ______________ Evening Phone: ____________

Employer/Source of Income: __________________________

Occupation/Work: ____________________________________

Education: ______________ Other Training: ____________

Special Aptitudes: __________________________________

Age: ____________________ Birth date: ________________

Marital Status: ____________

Drivers License No.: __________ Credit Card Type: Visa, Master Card

Credit Card No.: ____________________________________

General Health: ____________ Months since last physical exam: ______

Physical: ______________ Any notable findings: ____________

Please note any medication or other preparations: ____________

What specific problem or situation brings you in? (Summarize briefly.)

Here is a list of life-areas and common difficulties which often lead people to seek professional assistance. Please check those you feel may also apply to you. You may add any items we missed.________________________

Cohn - Visionary Quantum Healing™

What specific problem or situation brings you in?
(Summarize briefly.)

Name_____________ Date___________

Conditions You're Experiencing: (please check)

- ❑ Everyday Fears
- ❑ Residual Pain
- ❑ Guilt Feelings
- ❑ Alcohol Usage
- ❑ Artist's Block
- ❑ Anxiety
- ❑ Stress - Tension
- ❑ Sexual Dysfunction
- ❑ Phobias
- ❑ Post Traumatic Stress
- ❑ Childhood Trauma
- ❑ Smoking
- ❑ Insomnia
- ❑ Sleep Walking
- ❑ Motion Sickness
- ❑ Lack of Self Motivation
- ❑ Migraine Pain
- ❑ Low Self-esteem
- ❑ Energy-less
- ❑ Fatigue
- ❑ Addiction
- ❑ Relationship Problems
- ❑ Inner Child Rescue
- ❑ Uncontrolled Anger
- ❑ Head Pain
- ❑ Back Pain
- ❑ Neck Problem
- ❑ Heart Problem
- ❑ Lung Problem
- ❑ Liver Problem
- ❑ Kidneys Problem
- ❑ Blood Circulation Problem
- ❑ Body Contouring Problem
- ❑ Communication Problem
- ❑ Eating Problem
- ❑ Depression
- ❑ Drug Use
- ❑ Surgical Anxiety
- ❑ Work Problem
- ❑ Problem with Body Mobility and Functions
- ❑ Out of Synchronicity
- ❑ Rapid Aging
- ❑ Biomechanical Dysfunction
- ❑ Posture Trouble
- ❑ Other Conditions_________

____

____

Signature_____________

Cohn - Visionary Quantum Healing™

58. Client Agreement and Release from Liability

I, ____________________, agree to the following points of conduct during and after the course of my therapy.

* A fee of $______ is required to be paid in advance prior to any work for two visits 30 days apart if needed.

1. Appointments must be canceled at least 24 hours in advance.

2. There will be no refunds of any kind, regardless of results.

3. I will not use any mood altering substance (drug or alcohol) before coming to my session.

4. I understand—and it has been fully explained to me that—the types of therapies being used are exclusively alternative in nature, based on the whole-body healing philosophy: the integration of Body/Mind healing approach as a total being.

5. Energy, Chakras and Mobility testing sessions, if needed, require permission to touch the body at specific locations.

6. I understand that I am responsible for my well-being and healing process. The therapist can't "fix" or cure me.

7. The therapist reserves the right to refuse additional work and services to me.

8. By signing below, I agree and promise not to sue and hereby do release and hold harmless from liability and damages,____________therapist- practitioner from any and all losses regarding the above therapies.

9. I acknowledge that I understand the meaning of the above conditions by signing below.

Client: | **Practitioner:**
Name (print)______________________ **Name** (print)______________________

Signed______________ **Date**______ **Signed**______________ **Date**______

Clients/Members having any treatments must sign the Release & Consent Agreement:

59. Release And Consent Form

I _______________________ acknowledge that I have been advised and fully informed by __________ of the above noted treatment, including but not limited to possible complications associated with such procedures. I understand that __________ is relying upon the truthfulness and accuracy of such statements in determining which treatment is appropriate for me. I fully understand that the administration of the above noted procedure is not an exact science. I hereby confirm that no warranty or guarantee has been made to me covering the process or the results of the above noted process. I understand that there shall be no refund on any treatment. I hereby release and hold harmless __________ from and against all claims, demands, damages, costs, expenses and liability for injury or damage that may occur to me arising out of or in any way connected with the negligent performance of the above noted procedures. My signature below constitutes (1) my acknowledgement that I have read, understood, and fully agree to the foregoing Waiver and Consent, (2) the above noted procedures have been satisfactorily explained to me and I have all the information I desire, (3) I hereby give my authorization and consent to the above procedures, and (4) I accept the above terms.

Client:
Name (print)____________________

Signed______________ **Date**______

Practitioner:
Name (print)____________________

Signed______________ **Date**______

Appendix B:

White House Commission Final Report on Health and Alternative Medicine

"Now you know," an e-mail newsletter on health and alternative medicine, stated in a story on "The Natural Approach without Drugs or Surgery."

In March 2000, the White House issued Executive Order No. 13147, which initiated the White House Commission on Complementary and Alternative Medicine ("CAM"). The Commission was designed, for the first time, to look into non-medical health care. The Commission called all such care Complementary and Alternative Medicine (CAM), even though most of the forms of health care included in this category were not alternatives and certainly were not medicine in any form. Alternative Medicine was one of the CAM health care delivery systems included in the report.

In March 2002, this Commission released its final report. The Executive Summary of the report, published on its web site at http://whccamp.hhs.gov/, contained ten recommendations to be included in the final report. These ten recommendations, listed below, speak to very important and fundamental issues in health care.

1. A wholeness orientation in health care delivery.

   Health involves all aspects of life—mind, body, spirit, and environment, and high-quality health care must support care of the whole person.

2. Evidence of safety and efficacy.

The commission is committed to promoting the use of science and appropriate scientific methods to help identify safe and effective CAM services and products and to generate evidence that will protect and promote the public health.

3. The healing capacity of the person.

   People have a remarkable capacity for recovery and self-healing, and a major focus of health care is to support and promote this capacity.

4. Respect for individuality.

   Each person is unique and has the right to health care that is appropriately responsive to him or her, respecting preferences and preserving dignity.

5. The right to choose treatment.

   Each person has the right to choose freely among

safe and effective care or approaches, as well as among qualified practitioners who are accountable for their claims and actions and responsive to the person's needs.

6. An emphasis on health promotion and self-care.

   Good health care emphasizes self-care and early intervention for maintaining and promoting health.

7. Partnerships are essential to integrated health care.

   Good health care requires teamwork among clients, health care practitioners (conventional and CAM), and researchers committed to both creating optimal healing environments and to respecting the diversity of all health care traditions.

8. Education as a fundamental health care service.

   Education about prevention, healthy lifestyles, and

the power of self-healing should be made an integral part of the curriculum of all health care professionals and should be made available to people of all ages.

9. Dissemination of comprehensive and timely information.

   The quality of health care can be enhanced by promoting efforts that thoroughly and thoughtfully examine the evidence on which CAM systems, practices, and products are based and making this evidence widely, rapidly, and easily available.

10. Integral public involvement.

    The input of informed consumers and other members of the public must be incorporated in setting priorities for health care and health care research and in reaching policy decisions, including those related to CAM, within the public and private sectors.

From an alternative medicine standpoint, it is good to see these ten points being presented in such a public document. Many of the Commission's statements regarding wholeness, healing, wellness, and the right of the individual to choose his or her form of health care have been part of alternative medicine practices for decades.

The Commission recognizes the ever-growing role that non-medical care is having on the populace in the United States. In concluding, the Commission made the following statement, "the Commission recommends ... that the President, Secretary of Health and Human Services, and Congress create an office to coordinate federal CAM activities and to facilitate the integration of safe and effective practices and products into the nation's health care system."

The foregoing recommendations by the White House Commission help validate the work of the Visionary Quantum practitioner, who has long recognized the importance of holistic approaches to health and healing. The official endorsement of alternative medicine bodes well for future practitioners of this esoteric art of healing. Slowly, the theories and methods of alternative medicine are being accepted by the mainstream. The Visionary Quantum practitioner knows that the art is both learned and applied intuitively, and draws from the wisdom of generations. Thus, these practices must be regulated so that clients are protected from charlatans, and charlatans are protected from themselves.

Appendix C:

Case Studies and Testimonials

Case Study #1: Healing Other Healers

Lessons Drawn From Rimon Issac,D.O.

The beneficial effects of Visionary Quantum Healing extend beyond the simple cure of a particular ailment. In the case of Osteopathic Surgeon Dr. Rimon Issac, VQH helped him to such an extent that all of those interacting with him also benefited. The following is a photocopy of Dr. Issac's letter after his VQH session in the spring of 1998. Among the symptoms I detected in

Dr. Issac was an abnormality located in the left side of his brain that was affecting the spleen. He later acknowledged this malady, saying that he had known of it since his childhood and had sought the help of many doctors to cure his condition. None of them were able to detect the precise cause of his ailment, possibly because they lacked psychic vision.

Just as a car delivers better performance when it is finely tuned, so, too, with VQH; the benefits have a ripple effect. Dr. Issac speaks of psycho-emotional benefits in the form of increased "energy and vitality," "harmony in relationships," and "cheerfulness." Most importantly for him, perhaps, he also acknowledges that his "own healing power seemed to improve."

Testimonial #1

Rimon Issac, D.O.
Osteopathic Physician and Surgeon

5/10/98

To MR Salomon Cohn

Dear Salomon.

I want to thank you for your absalutely wonderfull Healing treatment last Week. I Came down with a cold on the Same day you Came to see me. I had high fever, sore throat and chills. Prior to that day I felt sluggish tired and had no Vitality. After your session was over I immediatly felt a charge in my energy and my well being. My fever broke one hour Later. after I went to bed I woke

up the next morning and to my amazement I was completly well from the flu symptoms.
For the following days I felt gradual increase in my energy and vitality. I want to tell you I just felt wonderfull, like a new man. My whole out look in life has Improved. My Relationship with my wife and daughter got anew Jump start. Your treatment was very deep and it affected me on many levels. In the psychoemotional aspect I was up, cheerfull and full of energy almost as much as I had ten years earlier. It also seemed that you touched me in other ways as well. I feel that you

helped me open doors that were previously closed for instance: my Relationship with my patients and my own healing power seemed to also improve. I was able to get to the Buttom of their issues and problems faster as if I could just zoom into it without any difficulty. I could cut through the layers of clouds that would have been there prior to your session.

I'm very thankfull to you for giving me the opportunity to meet you and be Blessed By the powers of healing you have. May God Bless you for many many years to come. And may you have the stamina and power and strength to contine this wonderfull healing work.

please keep in touch.

Sincereley,

Rimon [illegible]

Cohn - Visionary Quantum Healing™

Case Study #2 Francisco Alessi

In August 1999, Francisco Alessi called me for an appointment. He said he was referred by Bob, a dear friend of his and a client of mine. Bob spoke very highly of me. Francisco's first question was how much I charge per session. "One dollar," I replied, "for the full treatment."

"What? Are you joking?"

"Let me explain. The dollar is not for me. When you leave the session, and make your way home, give the buck to the first homeless person you see ."

Francisco asked, "How come?"

"I am doing research for the book I'm writing."

When Mr. Alessi came to see me, he sat on a chair and eloquently spoke of his symptoms. He was suffering from a bad back, bad knees, constant headache, and a sleep disorder, along with being overweight and a heavy smoker. I gave Francisco a Visionary Quantum Healing treatment. Mr. Alessi remarked that he felt much better after the session.

Just about a year and a half later, I received a call from Francisco. He was thinking of me and about how elated he felt. He wanted to again thank me for the marvelous treatment. During our conversation, I requested a favor: would he be good enough to write a testimonial about his past and present condition that I might use in my book? I thanked him for agreeing and bade him peace.

Cohn - Visionary Quantum Healing™

Testimonial #2

September 5, 2001

Hi Dr. Cohn,

For the past year and a half, since my friend Bob referred me, I've been thinking of you and telling all my friends about your magical healing. Thank God! I'm still amazed by the wonderful healing I got!

For the previous 10 years, I had been an impossible person to live with—a complete mess, both physically and mentally. I had a constant headache and I was not functioning at all. Always nervous and tense, I constantly fought with my wife and kids and everyone else. My family threatened to leave me unless I saw a shrink. I was suffering incredibly from my bad back and my bad knees. On top of all this, I was, as you'll recall, overweight, a heavy smoker, and suffering from a sleep disorder.

I want to thank you for your healing process. Your treatment was very deep. I want you to know that from that one treatment I have been transformed to a totally happy, healthy, and invigorated person. I feel great, both physically and mentally.

Thank you so much. My family thanks you, too!

May God bless you!

Sincerely,

Francisco Alessi

Cohn - Visionary Quantum Healing™

Case Study #3 Max Schlesinger

In July 1999, I returned home from an exhausting trip to Israel and New York. On my answering machine, the voice of my friend Judith Schlesinger implored:

"Salomon, where are you? Please call me as soon as you hear this message. It is urgent!"

The day I arrived home, I went to see Judith. She made a luscious dinner for her son Max and me. Max was on crutches. "What happened?" I asked. Max spoke of his trauma and suffering over the past five weeks.

"We've seen four doctors, and none of them know why my knees are swollen. I wanted to go to a traditional doctor, but they don't have any solution. Mom reminded me about the treatment you gave her ten years ago. You cured her chronic back pain. I hope you can help me."

I gave Max a single Visionary Quantum Healing treatment. The results were instantaneous; his pain and swelling abated; he could even walk without crutches. Four months later, I received a testimonial from Max Schlesinger thanking me, and telling me how wonderfully he is doing!

Testimonial #3

November 20, 1999

Dear Salomon,

I really want to thank you for your treatment in healing my knees. I went to see four different doctors and none of them knew what was wrong. My knees were swollen to the point where I couldn't bend. The doctors had no other solution other than applying pressure, icing my knees, and putting me on crutches for five weeks. As a last resort, my Mom finally got ahold of you. After dinner at our home, within the one single treatment I received from you, I felt so much better and my knees seemed to normalize. I was able to move my legs. As days went by, I was able to gain more movement in my legs, truly a miracle. I really want to thank you for what you did for me. I will never forget it.

Sincerely,

Max Schlesinger

Max Schlesinger

Case Study #4 Sason Gazel

In February 1998, Mr. Sason Gazel called to ask if I would please try to see him as soon as possible. His life, he feared, was going down the drain. He needed relief from his symptoms, which included extreme asthma and liver problems.

"Who referred you? " I asked.

"One of your clients, my friend David. He highly recommends you."

When Mr. Gazel came to see me, he sat on the sofa and spoke of his symptoms. He could not see himself coming out of the tunnel. His symptoms were nothing new to me. Since I mostly deal with difficult cases (physical and emotional), I knew that Visionary Quantum Healing was right for this kind of multi-faceted case.

After completing the successful treatment, I told Mr. Gazel that he should consider making some healthful changes to his lifestyle, including exercise and relaxation. Although 98 percent of clients require only one treatment, I told Mr. Gazel that if he felt that he needed one more session, he should not hesitate to call me in 30 days.

The last time I heard from Mr. Gazel, he was doing very well!

Testimonial #4

Cohn - Visionary Quantum Healing™

Salomon Cohn
1000 North Point
Suite 1103
San Francisco, CA 94109

May 8, 2000

Dear Dr. Salomon Cohn,

I am writing this note to you in appreciation for your gift of Visionary Healing and your professional services. I am happy to report that the condition I have had since 1982 is healed. I had extreme problems with breathing, asthma, my lungs and liver. It was so bad because I abused alcohol and hard drugs for nearly two decades.

I have been seeking professional help for many years and was told repeatedly that "I" was the problem. That's when I decided to come to you. Can you imagine my disbelief when you treated me with pure light energy — without even touching me!

I have been symptom-free since February 28, 1998.

I don't know what you have done to me. In just a matter of minutes — all of my sixteen years of suffering ended. Even my stress level has been completely reduced beyond anything I would have believed possible.

Thank you so very much.

Sason Gazel

Your new friend,
Sason Gazel
P.S. I love you — keep up the good work and may God bless you.

Case Study #5 George Benson

George Benson began his treatment on August 20, 1997. Referred by my client Nancy, Mr. Benson spoke of his "hopeless case" of chronic back pain. He had felt miserable for the past twelve years since a car accident in 1985. He had seen a neurologist and chiropractors, tried Chinese needle acupuncture, and various other kinds of holistic medicine. "I have done it all Dr. Cohn. Please help me out."

Following the first treatment on September 1, Mr. Benson continued to get better, and his condition became practically normal. Although most clients need only one treatment, in some cases the client may need a follow-up treatment. On September 30, Mr. Benson returned for a second treatment. At the end, George exclaimed, "Wow, I feel absolutely normal! Maybe this monkey is off my back."

George thanked me and practically danced out the door.

Testimonial #5

April 15.2000

Dear Dr. Cohn,

I have been thinking of you and telling everyone about you and your healing. You helped me out of the suffering and miserable condition that I had after my car accident in 1985. The treatment was marvelous and quick, with no disrobing, and without your touching me. I have been symptom-free since the last treatment I received from you on September 30, 1987.

Thank you very much,

Sincerely,

George Benson

Case Study #6 Mike Doty

I met Mike Doty in 2003 when I needed to help with a computer problem. I noticed his right hand seemed to be sore a lot while he was working on the computer. By healing Mike's hand, I was able to get three times as much work out of him!

After working with me for sometime, Mike was curious to experience the full Visionary Quantum Healing treatment. He had a sore foot and generally felt low energy. He also had some chest pain. Mike's aura was fragmented, showing a lot of blockage of the energy flow. After receiving the VQH treatment, Mike's aura returned to full bloom. A week after the treatment, his medical doctor checked the elasticity of his arteries as a measure of plaque and blockage using a new method called Cardiovascular (C-V) Profiling, developed by a researcher from Stanford University. C-V Profiling screens for susceptibility to cardiovascular disease and heart attack by measuring the waveform of the pulse to determine vascular elasticity, which in turn determines the amount of arterial blockage from plaque build-up. Mike's arteries were measured to be in the same condition as a typical teenager's. There was no sign of blockage. The sore foot got better and the chest pain went away.

Testimonial #6

Cohn - Visionary Quantum Healing™

October 15, 2004

I first met Dr. Cohn in September 2003, in response to a call to assist with a computer problem. I had a chronically sore hand from carpal tunnel, which was aggravated by working on the computer. Salomon noticed I was continually stretching and shaking my hand. He used his Visionary Quantum Healing treatment technique on my hand, after which the pain stayed away.

A year later, Salomon gave me one of his complete healing treatments. I had been feeling sluggish, tired, and had no vitality. After the treatment and in the days following, I reached a state of cheerfulness and energy comparable to what I had felt ten years earlier. My whole outlook in life improved.

The Visionary Quantum Healing treatment took place in Salomon's clinic. It took just twenty minutes. A week later, my physician ran a Cardiovascular Profiler test on me. My large and small arteries tested as being in the condition of a teenager though I am in my early forties. They tested the nerves in my foot for neuropathy and found no sign of damage. A few weeks later, I felt no more chest pain and my foot was back to normal as well. Thanks, Salomon, for the wonderful treatment. Keep up the great work!

Mike Doty

San Francisco, California

Case Study #7 Guy Gardocki

I met Guy Gardocki through a colleague in January 2003. He told me he had felt miserable for the past fifteen years. He had a fear of flying as well as other slight phobias. He had tried conventional and alternative self-improvement therapies for many years, without success.

In September 2004, Guy was visiting San Francisco on business. I met with him and gave him a five-minute treatment for a painful swelling on his arm. We also worked on his fear of flying. After returning to his home in Florida, Guy left an ecstatic message on my answering machine. He had felt unafraid flying home, and the swelling on his arm was gone. In general, he felt rejuvenated.

Testimonial #7

September 15, 2004

I visited San Francisco on a business trip in September 2004 and planned on visiting Salomon Cohn. I was introduced to Salomon in 2003. When I arrived at the hotel, I noticed extensive swelling in my right arm. The next day the swelling continued and it appeared that something had bitten my elbow, as there was a visible white mark there. I was an excellent athlete in high school and played college football at the University of Missouri. I'm familiar with injuries and healing periods as I have been active in athletics my entire life. My arm was not getting better and I even considered going to an emergency room. Monday I had several business meetings and lunch in the business district. I then went to meet Salomon to show him my arm and discuss my fear of flying. Salomon treated me for less than five minutes. Within two days, the swelling was significantly reduced. A week later, there was absolutely no trace of the swelling — amazing. Flying home from San Francisco to Miami, we experienced turbulence. With the seat belt sign illuminated and the flight attendants seated, I calmly watched the movie *Alamo* while we bounced around at 35,000 feet. Wow! Salomon has a wonderful technique. I have a spiritual base and have used alternative medicine and acupuncture before. Salomon's techniques work.

Sincerely, Guy Gardocki

Ft. Lauderdale, Florida

A.B.H.

Photo With The Legendary Ormond McGill

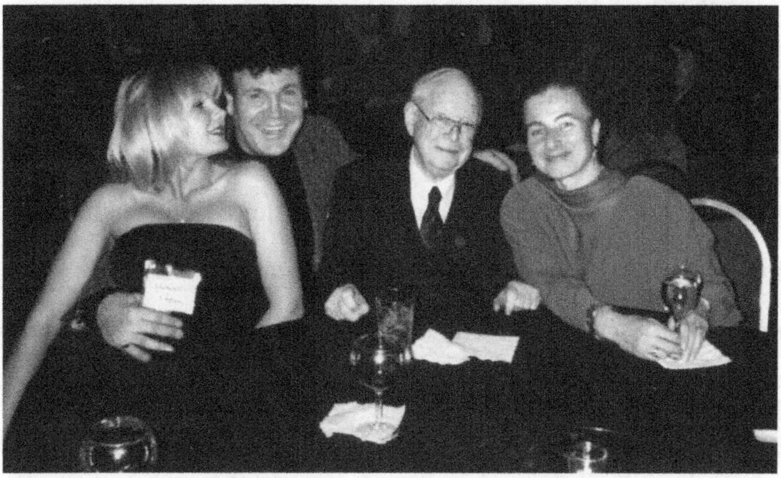

With great friends at the convention of the American Board of Hypnotherapists, Newport Beach, California, U.S.A., 1998, From left to right: Salomon Cohn, Ph.D. and a friend, Ormond McGill, renowned author and Dean of Clinical Hypnotherapy, and Marleen Mulder, C.C.H.T

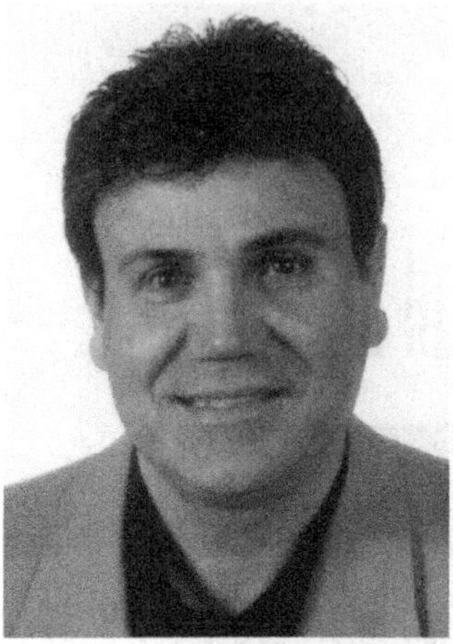

Appendix D

About the Author

Salomon Cohn, Ph.D., grew up in Jerusalem, Israel. He came to the United States in 1968, where his interests were, at first in family and business. As those two areas of his life flourished, he began to investigate a wide range of approaches that relate to healing and clinical hypnotherapy, the development of light and healing energy, biology, and human anatomy. In 1996, he earned his Bachelor's degree, a C.H.T. in Clinical Hypnotherapy, and became a Candidate for Doctor of Clinical Hypnotherapy, D.C.H.(c), at the American Institute of Hypnotherapy in Anaheim, California. He also studied at Harrington University in London, England, where he earned the degree of Doctor of Philosophy, Summa Cum Laude in Psychology in 2000.

Dr. Cohn is a member of the American Council of Hypnotherapy, an A.C.H.E. Examiner, and A.B.H. He studied with the esteemed Randall Churchill, Marleen Mulder, and Ormond McGill, known as "the teachers of the teachers."

Salomon has earned over forty certifications, including Clinical Hypnotherapy Practitioner, Feng Shui, Neuro Linguistic Programming, Time Line Therapy™, Reiki Master, Palm Therapy, Reflexology, and Deep Massage

Therapy. He is a Certified Voyager Tarot™ teacher and practitioner of Astrology, Metaphysics, and Graphology, Spiritual Psychic Reader, and a consultant/adviser using various tools for divination including Tarot cards, Numerology, the I-Ching, tea, coffee, and palmistry.

Salomon's wide-flung interests include becoming a certified piano tuner and repair specialist. He is a lay expert in antiquities, an inventor, collects art, paints, writes, and is a Certified Free Fall Skydiver. Memberships include Mystic Shriners (he is a Noble), Scottish Rite, and Freemasons NYC.

Dr. Cohn is founder of the revolutionary technique called "Visionary Quantum Healing," a healing method that facilitates one's inner physical and emotional well-being. He serves a national and international clientele, travels extensively, and speaks many languages. He specializes in difficult physical and emotional cases, including those with persistent pain, fear, and phobia. Most clients, after exhausting other resources, come to Salomon, a trend he intends to reverse with the publication of *The Complete Guide to Visionary Quantum Healing: 21st Century Healing for the Body, Mind, Heart, and Soul.*

In addition, Dr. Cohn has broadly expanded the number of his Visionary Quantum Healing seminars. An up-to-date schedule can be found at www.drcohn.net.

Dr. Cohn is the inventor of the $E=AC^2$ Duo Tech, a handheld healing device that diminishes pain and helps to restore a harmonious energy flow.

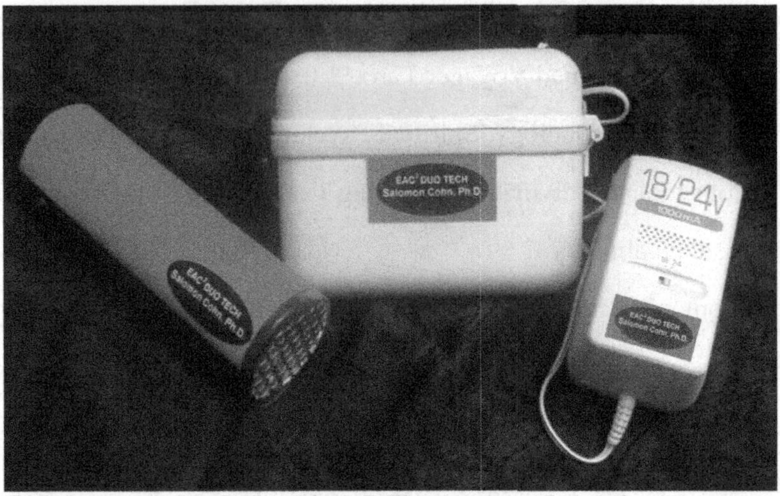

Electronic Medical Research: A revolutionary concept for the new millennium

The Body and Mind Prototype Curative

Disclaimer:

The following description is for an experimental device used for research in electronic medical experiments. We are not medical doctors or psychiatrists and as such we cannot make any medical claims nor can we prescribe treatment for or diagnose any ailment, illness or disease. Due to FDA regulations, we cannot make any claims as to what these devices will accomplish. We will be reporting on the results of our research in medical journals and on the Internet.

THE PROTOTYPE CURATIVE

A low-voltage earth-frequency energy wave generator, the E=AC^2 Duo Tech contributes to the field of non-invasive healing devices. It is a hand-held, pain-relieving curative operating at the Cohn high curative resonance frequency of seven cycles per second. Yesterday's science fiction has become today's reality.

Input: 110/220VAC, 50/60 Hz, 30w

Output: 18/24 VAC, 50/60 Hz, 1000mA

Rebalances the endocrine system and accelerates healing. The unit switches between low and high output.

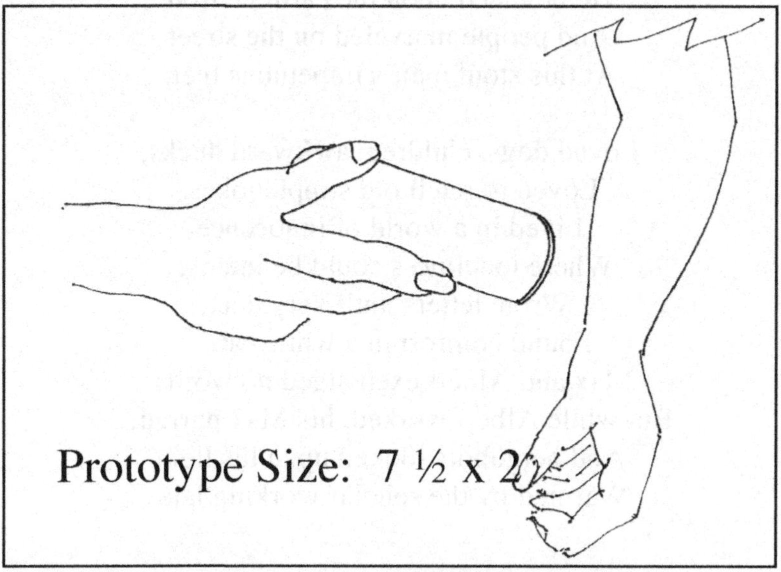

Prototype Size: 7 ½ x 2

Prototype E=AC^2 Duo Tech

Papa Albert

I have seen my father cold.
I have seen my father old.
His stride, purposeful, vital.
His talk struck from pure metal
Simple as gold, and all his learning
Only to light a passion's burning.
So beaming like a lesser god.
He bounced upon the earth he trod
And people marveled on the street
At this stout man's impetuous feet.

Loved dogs, children, awkward ducks,
Loved to retell old simple jokes.
Lived in a world of innocence
Where loneliness could be intense.
Wrote letters until very late.
Found comfort in a white cat…
Max and Albert exchanged no words,
But while Albert worked, his Max purred…
And neighbors looked up at his light
Warmed by the scholar working late.

I have seen my father passive.
He has been electrically massive.
He never hurried, so he said.
And yet a fire burned in his head.
He worked as an electrical engineer, for love.
And gathered in a world alive.
While black and white above his door
Spoke Mystery, the avatar…
A Hebrew inscription flowed
Like singing "In the name of God."

And when he died, he died so swift
His death was like a final gift.
He went out when the tide was full.
Still undiminished, bountiful.
The scholar and the gentle soul.
The passion and the life were whole.
And now death's wake is only praise.
As when a neighbor writes and says:
"I did not know your father, but
His light was there. I miss the light."

Dedicated to my dad, Albert Cohn.

Bibliography

These are books I have studied during the ongoing development of my philosophy of life and my commitment to healing with natural air and light energy.

Agnon, S.Y. *The Fiction of S.Y. Agnon.* Ithaca, New York: Schocken Books Inc. (1970)

Andreas, C. & Andreas, T. *Core Transformation: Reaching the Wellspring Within.* Moab, UT: Real People Press. (1970)

Austin, V. *Self Hypnosis: A Safe Self-Help Guide.* London: Thorsons, An imprint of Harper Collins Publishers. (1994)

Baker, A.M. *Awakening our Self Healing Body: A Solution to the Health Care Crisis.* Los Angeles, CA: Self Health Care System. (1994)

Bandler, R. & Grinder, J. *Reframing, Neuro-Linguistic Programming and the Transformation of Meaning.* Moab, UT: Real People Press. (1982)

Barral, J.P. *The Thorax.* Seattle, WA: Eastland Press. (1991)

Barral, J.P. *Manual Thermal Diagnosis.* Seattle, WA: Eastland Press. (1996)

Bourne, E.J. *The Anxiety & Pbobia Workbook.* Oakland, CA: New Harbinger Publications, Inc. (1995)

Brennan, B.A. *Light Emerging: The Journey of Personal Healing.* New York, NY: Bantam Books. (1993)

Brooks, W & Foss, N. *Breatharianism: Breathe and Live Forever*. Arvada, CA: Breatharian International, Inc. (1982)

Broughton, R.H. *Parapsychology: The Controversial Science.* New York, N.Y.: Ballantine Books. (1991)

Brown, C.P., Bernadeane & Strole, J.R. *Together Forever: An Invitation to Be Physically Immortal.* Scottsdale, AZ: The Eternal Flame Foundation. (1990)

Cheek, D.B. *Hypnosis: The Application of Ideomotor Techniques*. Needham Heights, MA: Pearson Allyn & Bacon (1968)

Chopra, D. *Quantum Healing: Exploring the Frontiers of Mind & Body Medicine*. New York, N.Y.: Bantam Books. (1990)

Cowens, Deborah, *A Gift for Healing*, New York, Crown Trade Paperbacks. (1996)

Ellsworth, P. *Direct Healing*. Glendale, CA: Westwood Publishing Press. (1982)

Gach, M. R. *Greater Energy at your Fingertips*. Berkeley, CA: Celestial Arts. (1986)

Gerber, R. *Vibrational Medicine: New Choices for Healing Ourselves*. Santa Fe, NM: Bear &Co. (1954)

Gerstein, L *Handwriting & Palmistry*. Potomac, MD: Nouvelle Press. (1994)

Gleick, James, *Chaos: Making a New Science,* New York, Viking. (1987)

Gordon, D. *Therapeutic Metaphors.* Cupertino, CA: Meta Publications. (1978)

Grinder, J. & Bandler, R. *Trance-Formations: Neuro-Linguistic Programming and the Structure of Hypnosis.* Moab, UT: Real People Press (1981)

Grof, S. *The Adventure of Self Discovery: Dimensions of Consciousness and New Perspectives in Psychotherapy and Inner Exploration.* Albany, N.Y: State University of New York. (1988)

Hall, Manly, *The Secret Teachings of All Ages.* Los Angeles, CA: The Philosophical Research Society, Inc. (1977)

Harman, W. & Sahtouris, E. *Biology Revisioned.* Berkeley, CA, North Atlantic Books. (1998)

Hass, E.M. *Staying Healthy with Nutrition.* Berkeley, CA: Celestial Arts. (1992)

Heschel, A.J. *Man is Not Alone.* Philadelphia, PA: Jewish Publication Society of America. (1951)

Huffines, L. *Bridge of Light: Tools of Light for Spiritual Transformations.* New York, N.Y: Simon & Schuster. (1989)

James, T. & Woodsmall, W. *Time Line Therapy and the Basis of Personality.* Cupertino, CA: Meta Publications. (1988)

Jampolsky, G.G. & Cirincione, D.V. *Change your Mind, Change your Life.* New York, N.Y.: Bantam Books. (1994)

Jung, C.G. *Alchemical Studies.* Princeton, N.J: Princeton University Press. (1970)

Kaptchuk, T.J. *The Web That Has No Weaver—Understanding Chinese Medicine.* Chicago, IL: Congdon & Weed, Inc. (1983)

Keller, Joyce & Keller, Jack. *The Complete Book of Numerology,* NY: St. Martin's Press. (2001)

Kom, E.R. & Johnson, K. *Visualization: The Uses of Imagery in the Health Professions.* Irvine, CA: American Institute of Hypnotherapy, (1983)

Laborde, G.Z. *Influencing with Integrity: Management Skills for Communication & Negotiation.* Palo Alto, CA: Syntony Publishing. (1994)

Laux, M. *Is "Modern" Medicine Killing You?* Potomac, MD: Naturally Well. (1995)

Leahey, TH. *A History of Psychology: Main Currents in Psychological Thought.* Englewood Cliffs, NJ: Simon & Schuster Company. (1992)

Lundin, R.W. *Theories and Systems of Psychology.* U.S.A.: D.C. Heath and Company. (1991)

Macrae, J. *Therapeutic Touch: A Practical Guide.* New York, N.Y: Alfred Knopf. (1993)

Mukrananda, S. *Kundalini: The Secret of Life.* South Fallsburg, N.Y: SYDA Foundation. (1990)

O'Brien, C. & Phillips, M. *Trance Formation of America.* Las Vegas, NV: Reality Marketing, Inc. (1995)

Orford, J. *Excessive Appetites: a Psychological View of Addictions.* New York, NY: John Wiley & Sons. (1985)

Ormond, M. *Encyclopedia of Stage Hypnotism.* Colon, Michigan: Abbott's Magic Novelty Co. (1947)

Oursler, W *The Healing Power of Faith.* Glendale, CA: Westwood Publishing Company, Inc. (1989)

Perls, F. *The Gestalt Approach & Eye Witness to Therapy.* Vancouver, B.C. : Aquarian Productions. (1973)

Phares, EJ. *Clinical Psychology: Concepts, Methods, and Profession.* Pacific Grove, CA: Brooks/Cole Publishing Company. (1992)

Robbins, T. *Jitterbug Perfume.* New York, N.Y: Bantam Books. (1984)

Robert, A. *Unlimited Power.* New York, NY: Ballantine Books. (1986)

Rosen, S. *My Voice Will Go With You: The Teaching Tales of Milton H. Erickson.* London - New York: WW Norton & Company. (1982)

Rossi, E.L., & Cheek, D.B. *Mind-body Therapy: Methods of Ideodynamic Healing in Hypnosis.* New York, N.Y: WW Norton & Company, Inc., Canada, Penguin Books. (1988)

Schlotterbeck, K. *Living Your Past Life: The Psychology of Past Life Regression.* New York, N.Y: Ballantine Books. (1987)

Scott C. *The Initiate: Some Impressions of a Great Soul.* York Beach, ME: Samuel Weiser, Inc. (1992)

Siegel, B.S.. *Love, Medicine & Miracles.* New York, NY: Harper & Row, Publishers. (1990)

Simonton, O.C., Matthews - Simonton, S. & Creighton, J.L. *Getting Well Again.* New York, NY: Bantam Books.. (1992)

Singer, I.B. *Old Love.* Toronto, Canada. McGraw-Hill Ryerson Ltd. (1979)

Small, J. *Becoming Naturally Therapeutic: A Return to the True Essence of Healing.* New York, N.Y: Bantam Books. (1990)

Smith, EE *Inner Bridges: A Guide to Energy Movement and Body Structure.* Atlanta, GA: Humanics New Age. (1994)

Spiegel, H. & Spiegel, D. *Trance and Treatment: Clinical Uses of Hypnosis*. Washington, D.C.: American Psychiatric Press, Inc. (1978)

Storr, A. *The Essential Jung*. Princeton, NJ.: Princeton University Press. (1983)

Talbot, M. *The Holographic Universe*. New York, NY: Harper Perennial. (1991)

Tesla, N. *My Inventions*. USA. Barnes&Noble Books. (1982)

Wang, R. *Qabalistic Tarot*. York Beach, Maine: Samuel Weiser, Inc. (1983)

Wanless, J. *Voyager Tarot: Way of The Great Oracle*. Carmel, California: Merrill-West Publishing. (1989)

Weinberg, G. *The Heart of Psychotherapy*. New York, N.Y: St. Martin's Press. (1984)

Wester H.W.C., & O'Grady, D. J. *Clinical Hypnosis with Children*. New York, N.Y: Brunner/Mazel, Inc. (1991)

Wilde, S. *Affirmation*. Sydney, Australia: Nacson & Sons Pty, Ltd. (1993)

Wilde, S. *Whispering Winds of Change: Perceptions of a New World*. Sydney, Australia: Nacson & Sons Pty, Ltd. (1993)

Whitehead, A. N. *Science and the Modern World*, New York: The Free Press, (1925 and 1967)

Index

About the Author, 19, 284
Acknowledgments, 4, 10
Addiction, 256
Affinity Energy, 91
Aftermath, 14, 145
Afterwards, 208
Alchemical Studies, 33-34
Alcohol Usage, 256
Alessi, Margarita, 5
Alternative Medicine, 7-8, 18, 251, 259-260, 264-265, 282
American Board of Hypnotherapists, 283
American Council of Hypnotherapy Examiners, 168
American Institute of Hypnotherapy, 284
Angels, 4, 16, 215, 218-219
Anxiety, 96, 246, 248, 256
Appendix, 17-19, 254, 259, 266, 284
Artist, 30, 115, 256
Astrology, 285
Atzeret, 155
Auschwitz, 62
Avi, 5
Awakening, 221
Ayurveda, 38-39
Back Pain, 256, 273, 277
Base of Spine, 91
Beautiful, 64, 165, 209
Beijing, 96
Beny, 5
Bhagavata Purana, 36
Biology, 27-28, 284
Biomechanical Dysfunction, 256
Blood Circulation, 256
Bloom, Dr. Richard, 15, 168-169
Body Contouring, 256
Body Medicine, 81
Body Mobility, 256
Bohm, David, 44
Bohr, Niels, 29
Book List, 23, 251
Book of Splendor, 110, 113, 165
Bordo, Mazal, 5
Breathe, 215
Brothers, 4, 62
Buddha, 166, 187, 191
Buddhism, 166
Burning, 286
Burst, 95
Butchers, 231
Celestial, 31

Cell, 172, 205
Center, 70, 90, 169
Century Healing, 1, 199, 285
Chakra - Crown, 91
Chakra - Heart, 91
Chakra - Ovaries, 91
Chakra - Third Eye, 91
Chakra - Thyroid, 91
Chemotherapy, 71
Childhood, 200, 256, 267
China, 98
Chiropractor, 4, 254
Chiropractors, 277
Child Rescue, 256
Childhood Trauma, 256
Chinese, 21, 49, 97, 231, 235, 277
Chinese Medicine, 21, 49, 231, 235
Chopra, Deepak, 15-16
Chronic, 94, 150, 196, 232, 273, 277
Chung, Jenny, 5
Clavicula Salomonis, 224
Churches, 254
Churchill, 284
Chutzpah, 112
Circulation, 256
Civilization,, 74
Claims, 245, 258, 262, 286
Clairsentience, 247
Clarification, 247
Clarifies, 113
Clarity, 4, 70
Classical, 94
Classification, 22
Cleansing the Body, 14, 139
Client Agreement, 17, 257
Client Information, 17, 23, 251, 255
Clinical Hypnotherapy, 218, 283-284
Cohn, Abraham Albert, 3
Cohn, Dr. Salomon, 206, 276
Coluccio, Mira, 5
Commanded, 36, 162-163
Commandments, 155-156, 162
Commandos, 152
Commands, 156
Communication Energy, 91
Congregation, 158, 162
Congress, 2, 264
Concentration, 13, 62, 126
Consciousness, 27-28, 34-35, 37, 74, 80, 84-86, 244
Consent Agreement, 258
Consent Form, 17, 258
Contents, 10
Copyright, 2
Cowens, Deborah, 47

Davis, 211, 220
Dedication, 3, 10
de Payrebrune, Mark, 57
Depression, 248, 256
Depth of Pain, 13, 121
Diagnosis, 21, 33, 70, 235-236
Difficult Cases, 20, 99, 236, 275
Disclaimer, 286
Dissemination, 263
Domain, 213
Drug Use, 256
Duo Tech, 285, 287
Duty, 167
Dying, 96-97
Dynamic, 30
Dysfunction, 256
Dying of Cancer, 96
Eddington, Arthur, 27
Eating Problem, 256
Efy, 5
Egypt, 7, 152, 156
Eidson, William, 56-57
Einstein, 25-27, 42, 70, 227
EKG, 75
Electronic Medical Research, 286
Elements, 221
Elena, 5
Elephant, 72
Elias, 5
Elie, 163
Elimination, 16, 140, 201, 251
Elisabeth, 28
Email Newsletter, 259
Embracing, 195
Emotional, 9, 20, 75, 79, 81, 91, 119, 180, 184, 196, 236-237, 250, 275, 285
Empathetic, 253
Employer, 255
Empowerment, 15, 186
Endocrine System, 287
Energy Field, 11, 26, 33, 47, 123-124, 126, 133, 236
Energyless, 256
Entity, 95
Environments, 262
Envision, 176, 197
Ephemeral, 37
Equal, 94
Equally, 153, 200
Equipment, 42
Establishing, 13, 126
Ezra, 153
Famous Master, 163-164
Fatigue, 248, 256
FDA, 286
Fear, 151, 168, 178, 196, 281-282, 285
Feng Shui, 284
Festival, 155

Film Director, 4
First Fruits, 155
Fish, Howard, 5
Fish, Judith Schlesinger, 4
Foreign Entities, 12, 31, 64, 76, 85, 119, 140-142, 145, 183, 203
Franco, 5
Frontiers of Mind, 81
Genesis, 11, 41-42, 101, 116
Gerber, Richard, 7, 26, 28, 80
Gleick, James, 7, 29
Graphology, 289
Great Healer, 224
Guided, 215
Guilt Feelings, 256
Hall, Manly, 87
Hand Healing Energy, 173-174
Hands of Fire, 58
Harvest, 155, 163
Hasidic Jew, 154
Hawaii, 206
Headache, 16, 22, 189, 201-203, 251, 271-272
Healing Began, 97-98
Healing Energy Link, 13, 126
Healing Hypnomeditation, 195
Healing Ourselves, 26, 28, 37-38, 69, 80
Heart, 1, 91-92, 178, 215, 248, 256, 279, 285
Heaven, 102-103, 114, 149-150, 166
Hebrew Calendar, 156
Heisenberg, Werner, 29
Bergson, Henri, 50
Hernandez, Ann, 5
Holograms, 44
Homer, 66
Homeo, 39
Homeopathic, 35, 38, 40, 63
Hovering, 130, 135, 139, 186
Human Anatomy, 284
Human Energy Field, 33, 236
Human Limb Regeneration, 15, 197
Human Services, 264
Hypnomeditation, 15, 23, 169, 191, 195-196, 221, 251
Hypnosis, 84, 168, 180, 188, 191, 195, 206, 246
Hypnosomatic, 82
Hypnotherapeutic, 169, 180
Hypnotherapist, 220
Hypnotherapists, 283
Hypnotization, 196
Hypnotic Induction, 186

Imitation, 14, 146-147
Improvement, 238-239, 246
Improvements, 246
Improving, 86
Improvisation, 171
Inanimate, 247
India, 7, 92, 146
Insomnia, 256
International, 2, 22, 285
Introduction, 10, 20
Inventor, 285
Investigative, 96
Israel, 60, 152, 165, 200, 208, 226, 273, 284
Israeli Military, 201
Jacob, 4
Jay, 4, 218
Jenny, 5
Jerusalem, 208-209, 284
Jewish Encyclopedia, 154
Joe, 5
Joseph, 5
Jung, Carl, 34
Kabbalah, 7, 49, 101, 105, 107, 109, 111, 155, 165, 245
Kabbalistic, 38, 87, 107, 160, 165
Kenny, 5
Kidneys, 256
Kilner, Walter, 52-53
King David, 14, 157, 159-161
Kingdom, 108
Kippur, 158
Kirlian, Seymon, 53
Kirlian, Valentina, 53
King Salomon, 159, 224, 226
Kirlian Photography, 51-58
Laser, 11, 42-44
Latin American, 96
Law, 17, 23, 40, 94, 199, 251, 254-255
Lawrence, D. H., 50
Legacy, 252
Legal, 2, 17, 180
Legally, 180, 254
Legends, 160
Legitimate, 229
Lesser, 42, 119, 288
Lesson, 113
Lessons, 94, 266
Letter, 24, 185, 254, 266
Levels, 8, 32, 76, 114, 180
Levy, 4
Lewis, 5
Liability, 17, 257-257
Liberated, 62
Libney, 152
Light Amplification, 43
Liver, 96, 189-191, 216, 257, 275-276
Magic, 62, 109-110, 223

Magical, 272
Magically, 160
Magician, 161, 224
Magnetic, 75
Magnetism, 25
Main, 102
Mainstream, 265
Maintain, 50
Maintaining, 262
Magnetic Resonance Imaging, 75
Marchelo, 5
Marleen, 283-284
Massage Therapy, 225
Maxwell, James Clerk, 25
Meditation, 193, 221
Meron, 165
Metaphysics, 218, 285
Migraine, 256
Miracle, 43, 103, 109, 163, 199
Mobility, 256-257
Moses Maimonides, 49
Moss, Thelma, 54-55
Motion Sickness, 256
Mount Sinai, 155, 162
MRI, 75
Multidimensional Negativity, 35
Mystical, 30, 161, 164, 224
Mysticism, 32
Mystics, 73
Nagasaki, 67
Nazi, 62
Neck, 144-146, 152, 183, 189, 252, 256
Nephews, 4
New Age, 80
New Choices, 26, 28, 37-38, 69, 80
Newtonian, 70, 80
Nobel Laureate Elie Wiesel, 163
Non-Medical, 8, 238, 265, 270
Non-Verbal, 20, 228, 250
Northern Galilee, 226
Numerology, 100-101, 244, 285
Orthodox Jew, 149, 154
Other Conditions, 256
Other Training, 255
Out of Synchronicity, 256
Pain Elimination, 16, 201
Palm Therapy, 284
Palmistry, 211, 214, 285
Papa Albert, 19, 288
Parapsychology, 247
Parks, Janet, 15, 179, 181
Passover, 155
Past Lives, 16, 224
Patients, 230, 241
Patricio, 5
Pauli, Wolfgang, 28

Pentateuch, 164
Perception, 75-76, 91
Persistent Pain, 285
Phase, 13-14, 22, 119-144, 251
Phases of Visionary Quantum Healing, 8, 13, 116, 118, 199
Phobia, 285
Pituitary Gland, 91
Poock, Gary K., 55
Post Traumatic Stress, 256
Protection, 14, 145, 195, 214
Prototype Curative, 19, 286-287
Psychic, 16, 48, 75, 91, 204, 210, 219, 267, 285
Psychology, 81, 284
Pure Light Healing Energy, 186
Purging, 45
Queen Isabella of Spain, 226
Rabbi Chaiim Pinto, 145, 186-187, 191, 224
Rabbi Ezran, 158, 162
Rabbi Shimon Bar-Yochaii, 15, 49, 163-165, 187, 190
Rea, Paul W., 4
Rosen, Paul, 5, 216
Rosha, Hila, 5
Schlesinger, Max, 18, 273-274
Schmidt, Joseph, 5
Schrödinger, Erwin, 29
Schurz, Dr. Jean, 5, 224
Shalem, Jacky, 5
Shamash, Elena, 5
Shlomi, Jewel, 5
Tobar, Helen, 5
Vibrational Medicine, 26, 28, 36-38, 69, 73-74, 80
Vital, Mony, 4
Webster, David, 5, 216
Whitehead, Alfred North, 27

Note

"In a moment of decision, the best thing you can do is the right thing, the next best thing is the wrong thing, and the worst thing you can do is nothing."

President Theodore Roosevelt

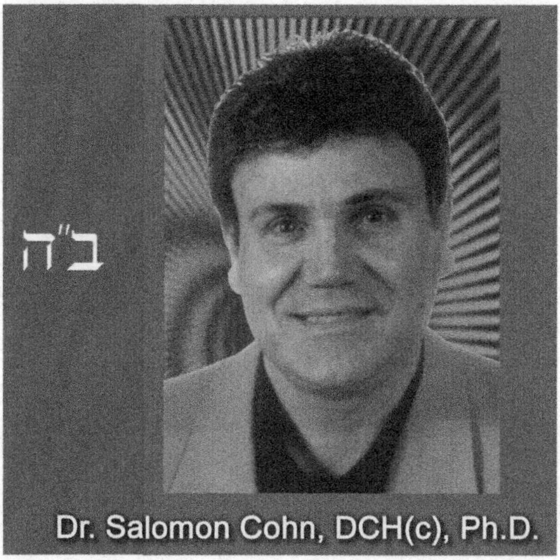

Visionary Quantum Healing works because it offers unified control of every organ in the human body. This is the ultimate noninvasive cure. It requires no belief system—only the suspension of disbelief.

Philosophical and scientific support for Dr. Cohn's method comes from Einstein's Theory of Relativity,Heisenberg's Quantum Mechanics and Rabbi Shimon Bar-Yochaii—as well as from other modern thinkers, including C.G. Jung, Elie Wiesel, Baba Ram Dass, Richard Gerber, and Charles T. Tart.

In this reader-friendly book, anyone can master Visionary Quantum Healing by following easy-to-learn steps that will provide instant healing. Illustrations and scientific theory provide additional support for learning the method quickly and easily.

Note

Made in United States
Orlando, FL
11 November 2026

90609404R00174